T0178115

Download Your Included Ebook Today!

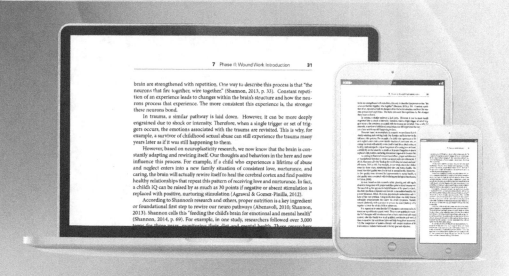

Your print purchase of *Biostatistics for Oncologists* **includes an ebook download** to the device of your choice—increasing accessibility, portability, and searchability!

Download your ebook today at:
http://spubonline.com/biostats
and enter the access code below:

1VLNTLUWR

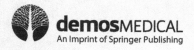

Biostatistics for Oncologists

Kara Lynne Leonard, MD, MS
Assistant Professor of Radiation Oncology
Alpert Medical School of Brown University
Providence, Rhode Island

Adam J. Sullivan, PhD
Assistant Professor of Biostatistics
Alpert Medical School of Brown University
Providence, Rhode Island

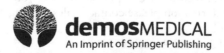

demosMEDICAL
An Imprint of Springer Publishing

Visit our website at www.springerpub.com

ISBN: 9780826168580
ebook ISBN: 9780826168597

Acquisitions Editor: David D'Addona
Compositor: Exeter Premedia Services Pvt Ltd.

Medicine is an ever-changing science. Research and clinical experience are continually expanding our knowledge, in particular our understanding of proper treatment and drug therapy. The authors, editors, and publisher have made every effort to ensure that all information in this book is in accordance with the state of knowledge at the time of production of the book. Nevertheless, the authors, editors, and publisher are not responsible for errors or omissions or for any consequences from application of the information in this book and make no warranty, expressed or implied, with respect to the contents of the publication. Every reader should examine carefully the package inserts accompanying each drug and should carefully check whether the dosage schedules mentioned therein or the contraindications stated by the manufacturer differ from the statements made in this book. Such examination is particularly important with drugs that are either rarely used or have been newly released on the market.

Library of Congress Cataloging-in-Publication Data

Names: Leonard, Kara Lynne, author. | Sullivan, Adam J., author.
Title: Biostatistics for oncologists / Kara Lynne Leonard, Adam J. Sullivan.
Description: New York : Demos, [2018] | Includes index.
Identifiers: LCCN 2017056849| ISBN 9780826168580 | ISBN 9780826168597 (e-book)
Subjects: | MESH: Biostatistics | Medical Oncology—methods
Classification: LCC RC267 | NLM WA 950 | DDC 616.99/40015—dc23
LC record available at https://lccn.loc.gov/2017056849

Contact us to receive discount rates on bulk purchases.
We can also customize our books to meet your needs.
For more information please contact: sales@springerpub.com

Printed in the United States of America.

To my family—Thank you for everything

To David Wazer—Thank you for your wisdom and encouragement in this and many other endeavors

Kara Lynne Leonard

Contents

SECTION II. IMPORTANT STATISTICAL CONCEPTS FOR ONCOLOGISTS

Preface

As a radiation oncology resident, I was often reminded of the importance of biostatistics in the study of oncology. An understanding of biostatistics is necessary for reading and comprehending published literature, for performing retrospective research, and for designing and analyzing prospective clinical trials. Biostatistical concepts are also tested on oncology board exams.

I noticed that, unlike radiation biology and medical physics education, statistics education was much less standardized. Biostatistics courses for oncology trainees are often taught by biostatisticians without a background in oncology or by MDs without formal statistical training. As such, many practitioners, both trainees and attending physicians, have a limited understanding of biostatistics.

I have had some formal statistical training as part of a MS program in experimental psychology. The MS program statistics courses focused heavily on experimental design concepts directly applicable to the biostatistics used in oncology. With this statistics background, I came to recognize that there are a few core statistical concepts critical to the practice of oncology. These concepts are repeated over and over again. To develop a comprehension of these concepts, I would pay careful attention when I read about them in newly published papers, and I would apply them to my own retrospective research.

The key, as I saw it, to understanding biostatistics in oncology was to focus on the core concepts and to apply those concepts to oncology-specific examples. I began to develop tools and mnemonics to share with my co-residents. As a junior attending, I designed a biostatistics course for radiation oncology residents in our program. I have been teaching the course annually for the past 4 years. The course has been well received, and residents have noted an improved understanding of sensitivity and specificity, categorical data analysis, and time-to-event data analysis. Residents have also mentioned to me that their scores on the statistics portion of the in-service exam have improved after taking the course.

In talking with my colleagues in medical oncology and surgical oncology, I learned that the need for basic, oncology-specific education in biostatistics was not unique to radiation oncology. Each specialty shared enthusiasm for a concise resource that simplified biostatistics concepts relevant to the field.

As I became even more aware of the need for an oncology-specific biostatistics text, I reached out to Adam, a biostatistician who focuses on education, and together, we created *Biostatistics for Oncologists*.

The book begins with the basic foundations of biostatistics that are tested on board exams (Section 1). In Section 2, these basics are then expanded on to include the concepts used in retrospective study design, analysis, and interpretation. The final section (Section 3) focuses on prospective clinical trials, guiding readers in their understanding of published clinical trials and in the design and analysis of novel clinical trials.

Most importantly, *Biostatistics for Oncologists* presents each concept with an example relevant to oncology. All examples focus on oncology-specific outcomes such as tumor response rate and progression-free survival. The section on Phase I clinical trials includes an example of radiotherapy dose escalation trials. The text also includes oncology-specific problem sets and oncology-specific multiple-choice questions for self-assessment and board study.

All of us in the field use our knowledge of biostatistics to read and evaluate published oncology literature. My hope is that oncologists reading a newly published clinical trial will reference this text to understand and evaluate the statistics section and, will use this text when developing an abstract for an annual meeting, or will flip through the book when developing concepts for new clinical trials. Hopefully, after reading this book, you will find biostatistics less overwhelming, more manageable and applicable to your practice, and even enjoyable.

Kara Lynne Leonard, MD, MS

GENERAL STATISTICAL CONCEPTS

I

Why Study Biostatistics? 1

WHAT IS BIOSTATISTICS?

Biostatistics is the application of statistics to the biologic sciences. Biostatistics is used commonly in medicine, particularly as it relates to medical research. Data collection, data analysis, and interpretation of results are all important components of biostatistics.

HOW IS BIOSTATISTICS USEFUL FOR ONCOLOGISTS?

Consider the following scenarios:

You are preparing for the your medical boards. You may have had some formal training in statistics, but you still desire a refresher as preparation for your exams.

A new randomized trial is published; it is potentially practice changing. Commentary suggests that the statistical analysis may have been subpar. After reading the publication, you do not fully understand why.

You have partnered with a pharmaceutical company to develop a Phase I clinical trial involving a novel oncologic agent. In writing the clinical trial proposal, you must work with a statistician to outline the statistical considerations and guidelines for statistical analysis. You wish to know where to start and how to communicate with the statistician.

In each of these scenarios, *Biostatistics for Oncologists* will serve as an excellent resource. The basic biostatistical concepts outlined in this text are tested on the medical oncology, hematology, and radiation oncology specialty board examinations because understanding these concepts is critical to practicing oncology. Comprehension of biostatistics is essential to reading and analyzing oncologic publications and to designing, performing, and analyzing retrospective and prospective clinical research.

Summarizing and Graphing Data

2

TYPES OF DATA

In oncology research and in biostatistics in general, data lies at the center of what we do. Data is the information gathered to answer a specific research question. The data we collect typically describes the subject, the intervention, or the outcome and is either quantitative or qualitative in nature.

QUANTITATIVE DATA

Discrete Data

Discrete data answers the question "How many?" or "What is the number of?" (i.e., how many prior lines of chemotherapy has a patient had, or how many distinct sites of metastatic disease does a patient have?).

Continuous Data

Continuous data is data that cannot be placed in discrete categories (i.e., age, tumor length).

As discrete and continuous data are both numerical, it may be difficult to distinguish the two. You need to ask yourself if certain values can exist. For example, consider the value 3.6. In a dataset that includes the variables age and tumor diameter, a subject can be 3.6 years old and can have a tumor 3.6 cm in diameter; these are continuous measures. However, the subject cannot have 3.6 distinct sites of metastatic disease – this would be a discrete measure.

QUALITATIVE DATA

Qualitative data (also known as categorical data) is arranged into categories and cannot be measured numerically. Variables are placed into descriptive categories that are ordered either nominally or ordinally.

Nominal Data

Nominal data consists of variables grouped into named categories. This type of data has no natural ordering and many times is ordered into either social or otherwise created categories. For example, subjects can be described and categorized based upon gender and race.

Ordinal Categorical Data

Ordinal data does have a natural ordering. For example, patients can be described and categorized based on a performance status scale.

Let us review the variables presented in a typical oncologic publication and identify the types of data they represent:

Variable	Quantitative or Qualitative	Discrete or Continuous	Nominal or Ordinal
Patient characteristics			
Age	Quantitative	Continuous when presented as age on a continuous spectrum	
Age	Can be presented as a qualitative variable if presented as age groups (e.g., 51–60, 61–70, 71–80)		Can be presented as an ordinal variable if presented as age groups (e.g., 51–60, 61–70, 71–80)
Gender	Qualitative		Nominal
Race	Qualitative		Nominal
Performance status	Qualitative		Ordinal
Tumor characteristics			
Tumor size/ diameter	Quantitative	Continuous	
Stage	Qualitative		Ordinal
Histology	Qualitative		Nominal
Regional lymph node involvement, Y or N	Qualitative		Nominal
Tumor location	Qualitative		Nominal
Tumor grade	Qualitative		Ordinal

(*continued*)

Variable	Quantitative or Qualitative	Discrete or Continuous	Nominal or Ordinal
Pain score	Qualitative		Ordinal
Number of metastatic sites	Quantitative	Discrete	
RPA class	Qualitative		Ordinal
Time to metastases	Quantitative	Continuous	
Treatment characteristics			
Toxicity type (e.g., cytopenia)	Qualitative		Nominal
Toxicity grade	Qualitative		Ordinal
Time from diagnosis to randomization	Quantitative	Continuous	
Radiation dose	Quantitative	Continuous	
Number of cycles of chemotherapy	Quantitative	Discrete	
Median follow-up	Quantitative	Continuous	

   Certain variables can be presented in different ways as different types of data. Age is inherently a continuous quantitative variable; however, it can be presented as ordinal qualitative data and even as discrete quantitative data.

Example

Age is often considered a prognostic factor in endometrial cancer with a poorer prognosis in older patients. Many of the trials investigating treatment of early-stage endometrial cancer group women into broad 10-year-age categories. For example, the PORTEC-2 publication (1) included age presented as an ordinal qualitative variable. In the patient and tumor characteristics table, women are grouped into the following age categories: less than 60 years, 60–70 years, greater than 70 years.

DATA SUMMARIES

MEASURES OF CENTRAL TENDENCY

We often summarize the data from a population or sample based on the center of the distribution.

Example

Let us consider the following example of a measure of central tendency:

If a study sample consists of patients with lung cancer, it will likely be important to record pretreatment lung function data. Let us imagine the study includes 20 patients with the following Forced Expiratory Volume in 1 Second (FEV1 [L]) values:

3, 3.6, 2.7, 2.4, 3.5, 2.5, 4, 3.7, 3.2, 2.3, 2.5, 3.3, 2.5, 2.1, 3.7, 2.5, 2.8, 2.4, 3, 2.8

Mean

The mean is the average. The mean of a sample $x_1, x_2, x_3, \ldots x_n$ is calculated by the equation:

$$\bar{x} = \frac{\sum_{i=1}^{n} x_i}{n} = 2.9L$$

The symbol $\bar{x}$ denotes the sample mean and the symbol, μ, denotes the population mean. For a full discussion of the distinction between the sample and the population, see Section 3.

Median

If you arrange the data from smallest to largest, the median would be the value at the center. By definition, half the data are above the median and half the data are below the median.

To find the median FEV1 (L) of the example data of patients with lung cancer, we first order the data from smallest to largest and find the center value or values:

2.1, 2.3, 2.4, 2.4, 2.5, 2.5, 2.5, 2.5, 2.7, **2.8, 2.8**, 3, 3, 3.2, 3.3, 3.5, 3.6, 3.7, 3.7, 4

Because this dataset includes FEV1 measurements from an even number of subjects, the median is the average of the two center values. In this case, the median is 2.8.

Knowing when to use mean and median may seem complicated and confusing. The mean is affected by outliers, while the median is rather robust to outliers. For example, if an additional FEV1 data point of 5.6 L was added to the preceding dataset, the mean would change to 3.1 L, but the median would remain 2.8 L. The effect of outliers is typically most obvious in the case of quantitative data.

If the data is normally distributed, the mean and median will be the same. If the data is non-normally distributed, there will be more of a difference between the mean and the median.

When dealing with a non-normal distribution of quantitative data or when dealing with categorical data with a large number of categories, the effect of outliers on the mean will be more obvious, as in the preceding example. In such a case, it may be informative to present both the mean and the median. If data is normally distributed, the mean is appropriate to use. In the situation where a quantitative dataset is characterized by a few data points at the extreme of the distribution (e.g., age of patients diagnosed with breast cancer), the median may provide the best measure of central tendency. With ordinal qualitative data for which the numbers have a quantitative meaning (e.g., pain score on a scale of 1–10), the data is often best summarized by the mean.

Mode

The mode is the value that appears the most often in the data. In the case of our example, this would be 2.5 L.

MEASURES OF DISPERSION

When summarizing data from a population or sample, we need information about more than just the center of the population or sample distribution – we also need to know how spread out observations are. Measures of dispersion help us understand the spread of data.

Variance

Variance is one of the most common measures of dispersion. Variance can be calculated with Equation 2.1:

$$\sigma^2 = \frac{1}{N} \sum_{i=1}^{N} \left(x_i - \mu \right)^2 \qquad (2.1)$$

With this formula, you can see that the mean is subtracted from each value in the data. To prevent a zero sum, each of these differences is squared. This squaring leads to having square units, which in most cases is hard to interpret. To bring the values back to their original scale, (i.e., FEV1, cm, years, . . .), we use the standard deviation.

Standard Deviation

The standard deviation is the square root of the variance and is displayed with the formula in Equation 2.2:

$$\sigma = \sqrt{\frac{1}{N} \sum_{i=1}^{N} \left(x_i - \mu \right)^2} \qquad (2.2)$$

Example

If we consider the previous example of FEV1 values for 20 patients with lung cancer, we can see that calculating standard deviation yields:

$$(2.1 - 2.925)^2 = .680625$$

$$(2.3 - 2.925)^2 = .390625$$

$$(2.4 - 2.925)^2 = .275625$$

$$(2.4 - 2.925)^2 = .275625$$

$$(2.5 - 2.925)^2 = .180625$$

$$(2.5 - 2.925)^2 = .180625$$

$$(2.5 - 2.925)^2 = .180625$$

$$(2.5 - 2.925)^2 = .180625$$

$$(2.7 - 2.925)^2 = .050625$$

$$(2.8 - 2.925)^2 = .015625$$

$$(2.8 - 2.925)^2 = .015625$$

$$(3 - 2.925)^2 = .005625$$

$$(3 - 2.925)^2 = .005625$$

$$(3.2 - 2.925)^2 = .075625$$

$$(3.3 - 2.925)^2 = .140625$$

$$(3.5 - 2.925)^2 = .330625$$

$$(3.6 - 2.925)^2 = .455625$$

$$(3.7 - 2.925)^2 = .600625$$

$$(3.7 - 2.925)^2 = .600625$$

$$(4 - 2.925)^2 = 1.155625$$

The sum of these values is 5.7975.

Then the variance of these is: $\sigma^2 = 5.7975\big/_{20} = .289875$ liters^2. We then find the standard deviation, $\sqrt{.289875} = .54$.

A low standard deviation indicates that the values in a sample are close to the mean, while a high standard deviation indicates the opposite – the values in the sample are spread from the mean.

Interquartile Range

Interquartile range gives a measure of data spread based upon dividing the data into quartiles. The interquartile range is the difference between the lowest number in the second quartile and the highest number in the third quartile.

Using the same example (FEV1 values for 20 patients with lung cancer) with data points arranged in quartiles:

1. 2.1
2. 2.3
3. 2.4
4. 2.4
5. 2.5

---

6. 2.5
7. 2.5
8. 2.5
9. 2.7
10. 2.7

---

11. 2.8
12. 2.8
13. 3
14. 3
15. 3.2

---

16. 3.5
17. 3.6
18. 3.7

19. 3.7

20. 4

Interquartile range = 3.2 – 2.5 = .7. The interquartile range works well with data that is not normally distributed.

STATISTICAL GRAPHS

Numerical summaries of data are crucial to research and understanding of data. Another aspect that is just as important for understanding data is the visualization of the data. Seeing the data visually represented in graph form can provide new understanding and perspective, as well as provide further details for the best way to proceed with analyzing that data.

We will explore some common types of graphs next.

HISTOGRAMS

Histograms display data in bar graph form (Figure 2.1). Histograms represent a particular type of bar graph that consolidates data with one box for each value (as opposed to one box for each data point).

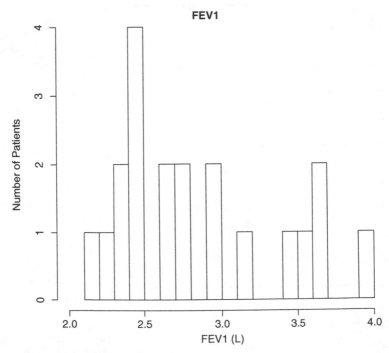

FIGURE 2.1 Histogram of FEV1 values.

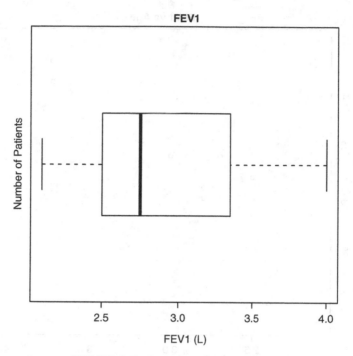

FIGURE 2.2 Box plot of FEV1 values.

Histograms are often used to display continuous data. The histogram allows for us to see the shape of the distribution of the data. Knowing this shape is crucial for understanding how to proceed with analysis.

BOX PLOT

A box plot depicts data through quartiles (Figure 2.2).

The thick black line represents the median of the data. The lines that fill out the rectangle are the 25th percentile and the 75th percentile. The other lines or "whiskers" represent the range of the lower and upper quartiles.

SCATTER PLOT

A scatter plot depicts data in two dimensions. For example, if we consider the ages of patients along with their FEV1 values, we would see the plot shown in Figure 2.3:

This graph displays an apparent relationship with FEV1 and age. Without this representation, it is difficult to find this relationship through numerical summaries alone.

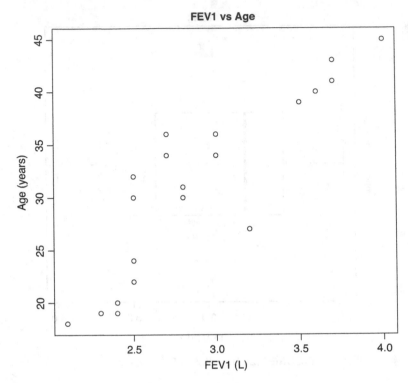

FIGURE 2.3 Scatter plot of FEV1 versus age.

REFERENCE

1. Nout RA, Smit VT, Putter H, et al. Vagina brachytherapy versus pelvic external beam radiotherapy for patients with endometrial cancer of high intermediate risk (PORTEC-2): an open-label, non-inferiority, randomised trial. *Lancet*. 2010;375:816–823. doi:10.1016/S0140-6736 (09)62163-2

Sampling

The purpose of research and data analysis is to study and make conclusions about a population. Examples of populations in oncology include patients with stage III lung cancer, patients with metastatic breast cancer, or patients who receive a new chemotherapeutic agent or radiotherapy with a novel technique.

POPULATIONS AND SAMPLE

Because it is often inconvenient, impractical, or impossible to study an entire population, a sample typically has to be chosen to represent the population. This representative sample is the group that will be studied to make determinations about an entire population. If the sample appropriately typifies a population, conclusions drawn about the sample may be directly applied to the population at large.

Example

Let us use an example from the Systemic Therapy in Advancing or Metastatic Prostate Cancer: Evaluation of Drug Efficacy (STAMPEDE) trial looking at the use of systemic therapy in advancing or metastatic prostate cancer (1). This study concerns a population of men with advanced or metastatic prostate cancer. This is an enormous population, and all men fitting this description cannot be practically studied. To represent this population, a sample of patients is enrolled. In this case, the sample consisted of 2,962 men enrolled at multiple participating sites. The men in the sample were randomly assigned to receive hormone therapy alone, hormone therapy plus zoledronic acid, hormone therapy plus docetaxel, or hormone therapy plus docetaxel and zoledronic acid. The primary end point was overall survival. Docetaxel chemotherapy, given at the time of long-term hormone therapy initiation, showed evidence of improved survival accompanied by an increase in adverse events. This conclusion is then extrapolated to the population at large and the authors recommend that docetaxel chemotherapy should become part of the standard of care for men in this population (those with advanced or metastatic prostate cancer) commencing long-term hormone therapy.

SIMPLE RANDOM SAMPLE

The most scientifically appropriate sample is a simple random sample. In the case of a simple random sample, each member of the sample is chosen at random and, as such, each person in the population has the exact same chance of being chosen for a sample. Such simple random samples are not practical and most of the time not even possible for trials in oncology.

Example

A feasible example of a simple random sample in oncology is as follows: An attending physician working with a second-year medical student wants to develop a manageable project for her. The attending physician is interested in looking at outcomes for all patients with stage IV colon cancer treated at his institution over the past 15 years. This population includes about 500 patients, and he would like to have the student review the records of a sample of 20%, or 100, of these patients. The attending physician suggests that the medical student choose a simple random sample to represent the population. He suggests that she enter all 500 patients into Microsoft Excel and then use the random number generator (RAND) to select the simple random sample, taking care that the same number is not chosen more than once. The data could then be collected on this more manageable sample to represent and draw conclusions about the entire population.

OTHER SAMPLING METHODS

After defining the population of interest, a sample must be selected. This can be done in a variety of ways. Other sampling methods include probability sampling such as systematic sampling, stratified sampling, probability-proportional-to-size sampling, cluster sampling, quota sampling, minimax sampling, accidental sampling, line-intercept sampling, panel sampling, snowball sampling, or theoretic sampling.

The most commonly used probability sampling methods in medicine are systematic sampling, stratified sampling, and cluster sampling.

REFERENCE

1. James ND, Sydes MR, Clarke NW, et al. for the STAMPEDE investigators. Addition of docetaxel, zoledronic acid, or both to first-line long-term hormone therapy in prostate cancer (STAMPEDE): survival results from an adaptive, multiarm, multistage, platform randomised controlled trial. *Lancet.* 2016;387:1163–1177. doi:10.1016/S0140-6736(15)01037-5

Statistical Estimation

4

The sample we choose represents the population we are studying. The cases in the sample may be spread out in different ways. This is referred to as a distribution. The characteristics of the distribution are important to the analysis of the sample.

SOME BASIC DISTRIBUTIONS

The following are examples of the basic ways that data within a sample may be distributed.

NORMAL DISTRIBUTION

Data that is distributed normally is a mirror image across the mean and has a histogram that looks like a bell shape. The normal distribution is also known as a Gaussian distribution. It is a continuous distribution and is widely used in research. Many biological variables, such as height, weight, and blood pressure, are normally distributed. Because much biologic data is distributed normally, a normal distribution is often assumed for other biologic variables. For example, in oncology, we may assume that a random sample of tumor size/diameter behaves like a normal distribution.

Example

Figure 4.1 demonstrates a normal curve created from age at diagnosis of 48 men with prostate cancer.

36, 37, 39, 43, 44, 45, 47, 47, 50, 52, 54, 54, 54, 57, 56, 55, 53, 60, 61, 65, 65, 66, 66, 65, 64, 63, 63, 68, 69, 70, 73, 74, 74, 71, 73, 74, 76, 77, 78, 84, 85, 86, 82, 81, 90, 91, 93, 94

The normal distribution is best described by its mean and standard deviation. The mean age of our example distribution is 65.1 years and the standard deviation is 15.3 years. With these two values, one can understand how

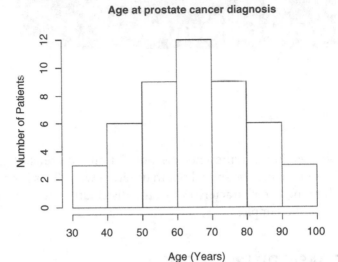

FIGURE 4.1 Age at prostate cancer diagnosis as an example of an approximately normal distribution.

the data looks if it is normally distributed. Within a normal distribution, 68% of the observations fall within one standard deviation of the mean, 95.5% of the observations fall within two standard deviations of the mean, and 99.7% of the observations fall within three standard deviations of the mean. In this example, 65% of the observations fall between 50 and 80 years and 99% fall between 35 and 95 years, respectively. This example displays a distribution that is very close to normal, but is not perfectly normal. This is exactly the kind of distribution you will encounter in research: something that is close to normal, but does not follow the theoretical distribution perfectly.

Central Limit Theorem

The *central limit theorem* is very aptly named. It is a theorem about the means of distributions, and it is at the center of much of the statistics discussed in this book and much of what you will find in oncology research.

Example

Let us consider the example of Forced Expiratory Volume in 1 Second (FEV1). FEV1 (L), values are collected from 20 patients:

3, 3.6, 2.7, 2.4, 3.5, 2.5, 4, 3.7, 3.2, 2.3, 2.5, 3.3, 2.5, 2.1, 3.7, 2.5, 2.8, 2.4, 3, 2.8

With this example, our histogram showed that this data did not appear to be normally distributed. The central limit theorem states that, if you took the experiment with FEV1 and ran this experiment many times, you would find that the means of these experiments follow a normal distribution. The benefit of the central limit theorem is that, if the experiment we are doing could be run multiple times over, we can assume that the means of the multiple trials of the experiment would be normally distributed.

Basically, no matter what the distribution of your data, the central limit theorem allows for the means to be normally distributed. Even if your data is categorical, the mean of this data would be normally distributed. For the means to be normally distributed, we need: (a) to have a sufficiently large sample size, (b) to have a variance that is not too large, and (c) for the mean of each sample to be close to the mean of the true population. These three criteria are not too hard to achieve; many times a sample size of 30 to 40 is sufficient.

Student's T-Distribution

The student's t-distribution is a family of distributions that look like the normal distribution. The student's t-distribution is symmetric and bell-shaped, but has longer tails than a normal distribution. The student's t-distribution is applied in a situation in which the sample size is small and the population standard deviation is unknown, in order to estimate the mean of a normally distributed population. The larger the sample, the more the shape of its distribution resembles a normal distribution. The student's t-distribution plays a role in the student's t-test (see t-tests in Chapter 5).

Standard Error of the Mean

The standard error of the mean symbolizes the variation between the means of different samples representing the same population. Remember that each sample is chosen (by any number of methods) to represent the population. The mean of the sample may not be perfectly representative of the mean of the population due to randomness. The larger the sample, the more likely the mean of the sample will accurately represent the mean of the population. If multiple small samples are chosen to represent the population, each sample may have a slightly different mean (again, due to randomness). The standard error of the mean represents the standard deviation of each of these means. Obviously, it is not possible to obtain data on all possible samples, and thus the standard error of the mean is estimated with Equation 4.1:

$$\text{Standard error of mean} = \frac{\sigma}{\sqrt{n}}, \tag{4.1}$$

where σ is the standard deviation and n is the size of the sample.

As the equation explains, the standard error of the mean decreases with increasing sample size.

Example

Using the preceding example of FEV1 (L) values collected from 20 patients:

3, 3.6, 2.7, 2.4, 3.5, 2.5, 4, 3.7, 3.2, 2.3, 2.5, 3.3, 2.5, 2.1, 3.7, 2.5, 2.8, 2.4, 3, 2.8

the standard error of the mean is the standard deviation divided by the square root of the sample size. In this case, the standard error would be

$$\frac{.54}{\sqrt{20}} = .12.$$

However, in a sample of 40 patients with the same mean and standard deviation, the standard error would be slightly lower at

$$\frac{.54}{\sqrt{40}} = .09.$$

Understanding the difference between the standard deviation and the standard error of the mean is important when considering statistical hypothesis testing. The standard deviation is a measure of the variability of values in the sample. The standard error of the mean is a measure of the variability of the sample mean, $\bar{x}$, and is a measure of the precision and accuracy of the sample mean as an estimate of the population mean, μ.

BINOMIAL DISTRIBUTION

In a binomial distribution, each event has two possible outcomes with a fixed number of n trials. One of the possible outcomes is considered a success, and one of the possible outcomes is considered a failure.

The binomial distribution is used when a researcher is interested in the occurrence of an event, not in its magnitude. For instance, in a clinical trial, a patient may survive or die. In this instance, the researcher would use the binomial distribution to study the number of survivors, but not to study how long patients survive after treatment.

Example

Let us consider the following example: A novel targeted agent is introduced for treatment of metastatic BRAF-negative melanoma. The drug company reports that, in Phase I trials, 10% of the patients taking the medication developed pneumonitis. In a Phase III randomized trial, this claim is tested. A total of 50 patients are randomly assigned to receive the drug. Using the binomial probability function, a researcher sets out to determine the probability that five of these patients will develop pneumonitis. Although it may seem counterintuitive, for the purpose of this calculation, consider developing pneumonitis a success and consider not developing pneumonitis a failure.

The probability of success (developing pneumonitis) is 10% (based on Phase I trials), and the probability of failure is, therefore, 90%. If the researcher would like to calculate the probability of five patients developing pneumonitis via the binomial distribution, the researcher would perform calculations according to Equation 4.2:

$$\Pr(X = x) = \binom{N}{x} p^x (1 - p)^{N-x} \qquad (4.2)$$

where N is the number of trials, x is the number of successes, and p is the probability of success.

In this example:

$$N = 50$$

$$x = 5$$

$$p = .10$$

$$\Pr(X = 5) = \left(\frac{50!}{5!(50-5)!} \right)(.10)^5 (.90)^{50-5} = .185 = 18.5\%$$

The probability for five successes (the probability of five patients developing pneumonitis) and 45 failures (45 patients not developing pneumonitis) is 18.5%.

Graphically, the binomial distribution of this example is shown in Figure 4.2.

POISSON DISTRIBUTION

The Poisson distribution is a distribution of counts. This typically is for a specific number of events in a given time period. For example, if you are considering the number of cases of pneumonitis that are seen at a particular

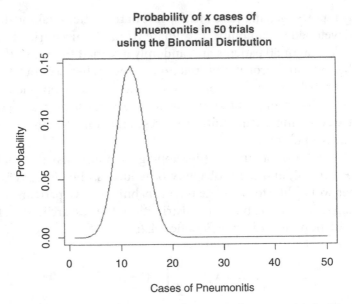

FIGURE 4.2 Binomial distribution of x cases of pneumonitis in 50 trials.

clinic over the course of one year, then you would use the Poisson distribution. Like the binomial distribution, the Poisson distribution again allows one to answer the question "what is the probability . . . ," but distinct from the binomial distribution, the Poisson distribution addresses the probability of success within an interval of time, space, distance, area, and/or volume. The Poisson distribution is also different because it typically gives the probability of a rare event in a very large or infinite number of trials. To utilize the Poisson distribution, you need only know the mean number of events within the given interval. In the Poisson distribution, the probability of events is given by Equation 4.3:

$$\Pr(x,\mu) = \frac{e^{-\mu}\mu^{x}}{x!}$$

(4.3)

where μ is the base or mean number of successes, and x is the number of successes in question.

In oncology, the Poisson distribution can be used to analyze cancer registries. For example, in a cancer registry, the Poisson distribution, which requires that malignancies be distributed homogeneously, is applied to identify geographic areas where certain types of malignancies may be increased (1).

Example

Consider the following example: Residents of a town note an anecdotally high number of leukemia cases, with 50 cases reported in the town over five years from 2010 to 2015. An epidemiologist sets out to determine whether this is the result of a true issue or the result of chance. On average, there were approximately 40,000 new cases of leukemia per year in the United States during this time period. This corresponds to 13.5 new cases of leukemia per 100,000 person-years. To determine the expected number of cases of leukemia in the town of 35,000 people being studied, the epidemiologist can use the Poisson distribution equation.

The goal is to solve for the number of cases in question (x).

Again, counterintuitively, consider each case of leukemia a success. The base number of successes is thus calculated:

u = 13.5 new cases/100,000 person-years
= .000135 cases/person-years

So, the mean number of successes is thus calculated:

x = .000135 cases/person-years × 35,000 persons
= 4.7 cases/year × 5 years
= 23.5 cases.

The mean number of cases in five years is 23.5. The probability of 50 cases of leukemia in five years is 7.3×10^{-7} and is most likely the result of a problem in the town.

See Figure 4.3 for a graph of the Poisson distribution.

In radiation oncology, the Poisson distribution is critical for two major concepts: (a) the number of decay events per time from a radioactive source, and (b) cell survival probabilities.

1. The number of decay events per time from a radioactive source.

The appropriate equation to model radioactive decay using the Poisson distribution is given by Equation 4.4:

$$\Pr\left(X = n\right) = \frac{(\lambda t)^n e^{-\lambda t}}{n!}$$

(4.4)

where n is the number of decay events, e is a mathematical constant, λ is the decay constant of the radionuclide, and t represents time. Together, λt is equal to μ, or the mean number of events.

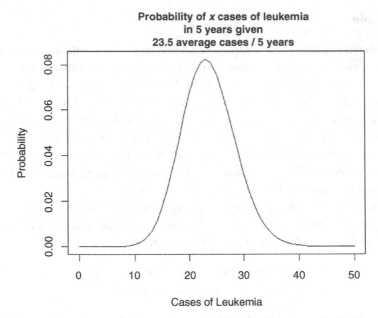

FIGURE 4.3 Poisson distribution of the probability of *x* cases of leukemia in five years given $\mu = 23.5$ (average number of cases in five years).

Example

The radioactive decay per year of ^{60}Co with a half-life $(t_{1/2})$ of 5.27 years would look like:

$$\lambda = \frac{\ln(2)}{5.27} = .132/year$$

So, for one year, the average number of events is:

$$\mu = \lambda t = .132/year \times 1\ year = .132$$

We can view the probability of decay in this example as shown graphically in Figure 4.4.

Example

Take, for example, a radiation oncology department installing a new stereotactic radiosurgery unit composed of multiple ^{60}Co sources. The decay constant of ^{60}Co is .132 per year. Implicit in the cost of the unit is the expectation that the sources will have to be changed at some interval. The administration would like to know the probability of decay in 10 years.

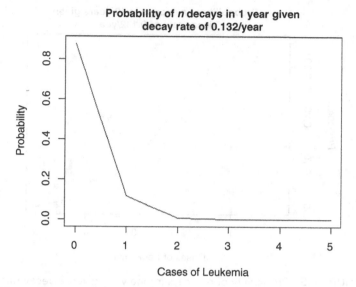

FIGURE 4.4   Probability of n decays in one year, given λ decay rate.

The following calculations would follow:

$$\lambda = \frac{\ln(2)}{5.27} = .132/year$$

So, over a 10-year period, the average number of events will be:

$$\mu = \lambda t = .132/\text{year} \times 10 \; years = 1.32$$

The radioactive decay over 10 years of ^{60}Co with a half-life ($t_{1/2}$) of 5.27 years is visible in Figure 4.5.

Radioactive decay is more simply modeled by the following equation of exponential decay (Equation 4.5):

$$Nt = N_0 e^{-\lambda t} \tag{4.5}$$

where N_0 is the initial activity of a radioactive substance, e is a mathematical constant, λ is the decay constant radionuclide, and t represents time.

Let us consider the same department installing a new stereotactic radiosurgery unit composed of multiple ^{60}Co sources that each has initial activity of 200 Ci. The half-life ($t_{1/2}$) of ^{60}Co is 5.27 years. The administration will not agree to exchange the sources sooner than 10 years from the installation date. The administration asks the physics department to calculate what the activity of each of these sources will be in 10 years.

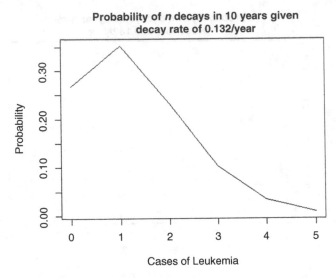

FIGURE 4.5 Probability of n decays in one year, given λ decay rate.

The calculation would start by calculating μ:

$$\mu = -\lambda t$$

$$\lambda = \frac{\ln(2)}{5.27 \ years} = .132/year$$

$$t = 10 \ years$$

$$\mu = -\lambda t = .132/year \times 10 \ years = -1.32$$

We expect that activity of the remaining source to be $e^{-1.32} = .267$ of the original activity.

$$200 \ Ci \times .267 = 53.4 \ Ci \ remaining.$$

The decay function using the exponential decay distribution is visible in Figure 4.6.

2. Cell survival probabilities

Example

Imagine you are irradiating a known number of cells in a petri dish. If each "hit" or double-stranded DNA break from radiation is assumed to result in

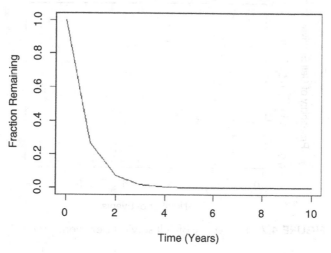

Fraction remaining at time (t) as a function of exponential decay

FIGURE 4.6 Fraction remaining at time (t) as a function of exponential decay.

cell inactivation, then the probability of survival is the probability of not being hit with a double-stranded DNA break.

The appropriate equation to model cell survival using the Poisson distribution is Equation 4.6:

$$\Pr(x,\mu) = \frac{e^{-\mu}\mu^{x}}{x!} \tag{4.6}$$

where μ is the average number of hits that occur and x is the specific number of hits.

So, to calculate the probability of a cell surviving a hit ($x = 0$ because in order for the cell to survive, it would experience no events) when the average number of events is 1 ($\mu = 1$):

$$\Pr(x,\mu) = \frac{e^{-\mu}\mu^{x}}{x!} = \frac{e^{-1}1^{0}}{0!} = \frac{.37 \times 1}{1} = .37.$$

The probability of cell survival in this scenario is, therefore, .37 or 37%. This logic and equation is often used to identify the mean lethal dose (D_{0}), or the dose that delivers on average, one lethal event per target and results in 37% survival.

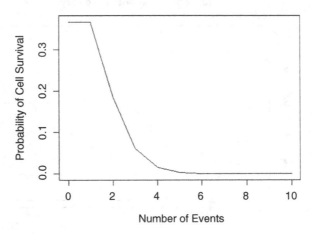

FIGURE 4.7   Probability of cell survival per event for $\mu = 1$

The cell survival curve governed by the Poisson distribution is visible in Figure 4.7.

As the radiation dose increases, the probability of survival decreases by Equation 4.7:

$$\frac{N}{N_0} = 1 - \left(1 - e^{-D/D_0}\right)^n \tag{4.7}$$

where D = the treatment dose, D_0 is the mean lethal dose as discussed, and n is a parameter known as the extrapolation number (which we will assume to be 1).

If you know that a single fraction of five Gy results in survival of 37% of the cells, what percentage of cells would you expect to survive after a single dose of 18 Gy (again, assume the extrapolation number = 1)?

$$D = 18 \text{ Gy}$$

$$D_0 = 5 \text{ Gy}$$

$$n = 1$$

Surviving fraction = $1 - (1 - e^{-D/D_0})^n = .027$ or 2.7%.

See Figure 4.8 for how cell survival for this scenario is represented graphically.

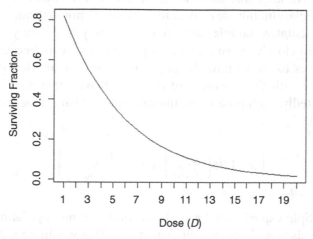

FIGURE 4.8 Surviving fraction as a function of dose for $D_0 = 5$ Gy.

ESTIMATION

Estimation is what we do when we do not know the actual value of a specific parameter. For example, in the normal distribution, we have two parameters: the mean and the standard deviation. We may use the sample mean to estimate the true mean. We have two types of estimators that we utilize: point and interval estimates.

POINT ESTIMATES

A point estimate is a single value used to estimate an unknown parameter. This would be the case of using the sample mean to represent the population mean. This also could be where we take a sample of subjects and look at how many of them develop pneumonitis. Then, we could use this proportion to represent the probability of developing pneumonitis in the population.

INTERVAL ESTIMATES

Interval estimates are many times preferred to point estimates. We discussed in the section on Normal Distribution that the sample mean is normally distributed. This means a simple point estimate is not able to describe the entire distribution. A range of values possible for the mean might prove to be more useful.

A confidence interval is a range of values used to estimate an unknown parameter. We are most often using biostatistics to make a conclusion about a population, but we cannot test the entire population, so we must use a representative sample. But, we have no way to be truly sure that a sample mean closely approximates the population mean, because there is no way for us to truly know the population mean. Confidence intervals work closely with the central limit theorem. If we performed an experiment repeatedly, each time we would calculate a mean. If we then created the interval:

$$\left(\bar{x}-1.96\left(\sigma/\sqrt{n}\right),\bar{x}+1.96\left(\sigma/\sqrt{n}\right)\right)$$

in multiple experimental samples from the same population, 95% of these intervals would contain the true mean. This would be a 95% confidence interval. A common misconception is that this means we are 95% confident that the mean is contained in this interval. However, the 95% confidence actually means that, if we constructed the intervals in this way each time, 95% of them would contain the population mean. Another way of thinking about this would be that, if we took 100 different samples of the population and constructed the interval above, 95 of those intervals would contain the true population mean.

Example

Although examples here are not very practical, an example may help illustrate the concept of confidence intervals. If the population we want to study is all patients with stage IV carcinoma, the population is so large that it would be impossible to study the entire population. We want to understand the mean age of patients with stage IV cancer. If we take a sample of, for example, 20 patients, with a mean age of 59 years and a standard deviation of 9, we might not have a lot of confidence that this sample contains the population mean. Then, we take 19 more samples (for a total of 20 samples). From each sample of 20 patients, we calculate a 95% confidence interval:

$$\left(\bar{x}-1.96\left(\sigma/\sqrt{n}\right),\bar{x}+1.96\left(\sigma/\sqrt{n}\right)\right)$$

In total, 19 of these 20 intervals would contain the true mean age of all patients with stage IV cancer.

Equation 4.8 demonstrate the formula to calculate confidence intervals for a sample:

$$CI = \bar{x} \pm z^* \left(\frac{\sigma}{\sqrt{n}} \right) \qquad (4.8)$$

The value of z for each respective confidence interval is as follows:

Confidence interval	z value
99%	2.58
95%	1.96
90%	1.645

For the example of a sample of 20 patients with a mean age of 59 and a standard deviation of 9, to calculate the 95% confidence intervals:

$$\text{Mean} = 59$$

$$\text{Std. Error of Mean (EM)} = \frac{\sigma}{\sqrt{n}} = \frac{9}{\sqrt{20}} = 2.01$$

We can use the previous sample to demonstrate how to calculate the 99%, 95%, and 90% confidence intervals for the sample:

99% CI = 59 ± (2.58 × 2.01) = 59 ± 5.19 = (53.81, 64.19)

95% CI = 59 ± (1.96 × 2.01) = 59 ± 3.94 = (55.06, 62.94)

90% CI = 59 ± (1.645 × 2.01) = 59 ± 3.31 = (55.69, 62.31)

Confidence interval estimations are very important in hypothesis testing, as discussed in Chapter 5, in the section entitled Confidence Intervals and Hypothesis Tests: How Are They Related?

REFERENCE

1. Westermeier T, Michaelis J. Applicability of the Poisson distribution to model the data of the German Children's Cancer Registry. *Radiat Environ Biophys*. 1995;34:7–11.

Section I Problem Set

1. The following is a table of patient characteristics presented in a publication of a hypothetical oncology clinical trial. Appropriately describe each of the variables as quantitative or qualitative. If quantitative, further describe whether the variable is presented as discrete or continuous. If qualitative, further describe whether the variable is presented as nominal or ordinal.

Variable	Group A n = 105 n (%)	Group B n = 103 n (%)
Age in years (mean)	65	65
Age		
<60	52(50)	49(48)
≥60	53(50)	54(52)
Gender		
M	50(48)	53(51)
F	55(52)	50(49)
KPS		
100	41(39)	37(36)
90	47(45)	58(56)
80	12(11)	5(5)
70	5(5)	3(3)
Primary tumor site		
Lung	38(36)	28(27)
Breast	21(20)	27(26)
Colon	29(28)	28(27)

(continued)

Variable	Group A n = 105 n (%)	Group B n = 103 n (%)
Prostate	17(16)	20(19)
Primary tumor diameter in cm (mean)	2.7	2.9
T stage		
T1	25(24)	30(29)
T2	40(38)	51(50)
T3	32(30)	19(18)
T4	8(8)	3(3)
N stage		
N1	57(54)	49(48)
N2	33(31)	37(36)
N3	15(14)	17(17)
Number of metastatic sites	7	10
Number of painful sites		
Single = 1	33(31)	41(40)
Multiple >1	72(69)	62(60)
Serum Hgb (mean)	10.8	11.1
Serum Hgb		
Normal	25(24)	19(18)
Abnormal	80(76)	84(82)
Marital status		
Single	63(60)	67(65)
Married	42(40)	36(35)

2. The following is a list of outcomes that is being investigated in the same hypothetical clinical trial. Appropriately describe each of the variables as quantitative or qualitative. If quantitative, further describe whether the variable is presented as discrete or continuous. If qualitative, further describe whether the variable is presented as nominal or ordinal.

Variable	Group A n = 105 n (%)	Group B n = 103 n (%)
Number of patients developing adverse effect	11(10)	18(17)
Response rate		
No response	41(39)	33(32)
Partial response	35(33)	45(44)
Complete response	29(28)	25(24)
Survival		
Alive	77(73)	90(87)
Dead	28(27)	13(13)
Median survival (mos)	26 months	33 months
Acute toxicity		
Grade 1	25(24)	33(32)
Grade 2	13(12)	19(18)
Grade 3	10(10)	15(15)
Grade 4	0(0)	0(0)

3. We have a sample of patients with Hodgkin's lymphoma chosen to represent a population of patients with the same disease in a clinical trial. In order to be included, patients had to have stage I to II Hodgkin's lymphoma and be 20 to 75 years of age. There are a total of 360 patients included in the study. The mean age of the sample is 39 years and the median age is 36 years. The age of patients in the study ranges from 21 to 73 years and the distribution is left-skewed. There are some outliers of older patients.

The data is presented in Table 1 of the paper, as follows:

Variable	All Patients
Age (mean +/− SD)	39 +/− 14

a. What is the relative disadvantage of using mean age as opposed to median age as a measure of central tendency of the age of the patients in this sample?

b. Which measure of dispersion would be most appropriate to describe how much the ages of individuals within the sample differ from the mean age of the sample?

c. Calculate the standard error of the mean (SEM).

d. What does the standard error of the mean represent?

e. How does the standard error of the mean compare if you have a sample size of $n = 100$ versus $n = 360$?

f. Imagine that the sample is normally distributed. What age range would include the ages of 95% of the patients? What age range would include the ages of 67% of the patients?

4. What are the mean, median, and mode of the following dataset?

290, 745, 678, 892, 320, 593, 360, 483, 494, 538, 487, 360, 279, 811, 736, 593, 479

5. Clinical trials have shown that the response rate (probability of at least partial response) with a novel immunotherapy agent in patients with metastatic non-small cell lung cancer with PD-L1 overexpression is approximately 40%. A cancer center anticipates treating 100 such patients with this agent, and the physicians want to determine the probability that 50 of these patients will have a response. Answer the following questions using the binomial distribution.

a. What is the probability of success (response) with this treatment?

b. What is the probability of failure (no response) with this treatment?

c. What is the number of trials?

d. What is the number of successes (x)?

e. What is the probability that 50 of these patients will have a response?

6. Research has shown that stomach cancer occurs in men in the United States at an incidence rate of approximately six per 100,000 person-years. Using a Poisson distribution model, what is the probability of one case of stomach cancer developing in 100 U.S. person-years?

a. Using a Poisson distribution, what is the number of successes in question (x)?

b. Using a Poisson distribution, what is the mean/base number of successes (u)?

c. Using a Poisson distribution model, what is the probability of one case of stomach cancer developing in 100 U.S. person-years?

d. Using a binomial distribution, what is the number of trials (n)?

e. Using a binomial distribution, what is the number of successes (x)?

f. Using the binomial distribution, what is the probability of success (probability of developing gastric cancer in this case)?

g. Using a binomial distribution, what is the probability of one case of stomach cancer developing in 100 U.S. person-years?

7. You are testing the radiosensitivity of cells in culture. You plate the cells and then irradiate them with varying single-fraction treatments. From your prior studies with the same cell line, you know that a single fraction of two Gy results in survival of 37% of the cells. What percentage of cells would you expect to survive after a single dose of 10 Gy? (Assume the extrapolation number = 1.)

   a. What is the value of D?
   b. What is the value of D_0?
   c. What is the surviving fraction?

8. A Phase III clinical trial is conducted to test a novel immuno-therapy agent in stage IV non-small cell lung cancer (NSCLC). Inclusion criteria allow patient's age 18 to 75 years with stage IV NSCLC without brain metastases who have failed first-line chemotherapy to be included in the trial. A sample of 300 patients is intended to be enrolled. The intention is for this sample to be representative of the population of all patients with stage IV NSCLC who have failed first-line chemotherapy agents. The mean age of the sample is 65 years, the standard deviation is 9.4 years.

   a. What is the 95% confidence interval for age?
   b. If you were to take 20 similar samples all of which have means that fall within the 95% confidence interval, how many of these intervals would you expect to include the population mean?

Section I Problem Set Solutions

1.

Variable	Quantitative or Qualitative	Discrete or Continuous	Nominal or Ordinal
Age presented as mean	Quantitative	Continuous	
Age presented as <60 and ≥60	Qualitative		Ordinal
Gender	Qualitative		Nominal
KPS	Qualitative		Ordinal
Primary tumor site	Qualitative		Nominal
Primary tumor diameter in cm (mean)	Quantitative	Continuous	
T stage	Qualitative		Ordinal
N stage	Qualitative		Ordinal
Number of metastatic sites	Quantitative	Discrete	
Number of painful sites	Qualitative		Nominal
Single = 1			
Multiple >1			
Serum hemoglobin presented as mean	Quantitative	Continuous	
Serum hemoglobin presented as normal vs. abnormal	Qualitative		Nominal
Marital status	Qualitative		Nominal

2.

Variable	Quantitative or Qualitative	Discrete or Continuous	Nominal or Ordinal
Number of patients developing adverse effect	Quantitative	Discrete	
Response rate presented as NR, PR, or CR	Qualitative		Nominal
Survival presented as dead or alive	Qualitative		Nominal
Median survival (mos)	Quantitative	Continuous	
Acute toxicity grade	Qualitative		Ordinal

3.

a. The mean is dramatically affected by outliers

b. Standard deviation

c. $\text{SEM} = \dfrac{\text{standard deviation}}{\sqrt{n}} = \dfrac{14}{\sqrt{360}} = .738$

d. Standard error of the mean (SEM)

e. Larger

$$\text{SEM} = \dfrac{\text{standard deviation}}{\sqrt{n}} = \dfrac{14}{\sqrt{100}} = 1.4$$

$$\text{SEM} = \dfrac{\text{standard deviation}}{\sqrt{n}} = \dfrac{14}{\sqrt{360}} = .738$$

f. The age range that includes the ages of 95% of m = 11 to 67 years

The age range that includes the ages of 67% of m = 25 to 53 years

4.

Mean = 538
Median = 494
Mode = 593, 360 (both appear twice)

5.

    a. Probability of success = 40%

    b. Probability of failure = 60%

    c. Number of trials = 100

    d. Number of successes = 50

    e. $P = \binom{N}{x} p^x (1-p)^{N-x}$

    Probability that 50 patients will have a response:

    $P(x = 50) = (100!/(50!) \times (100 - 50)!)(0.4)^{100}(0.6)^{100-50} = .010$

6.

    a. Number of successes $(x) = 1$

    b. Mean/Base number of successes $(u) =$

            = (incidence rate) × (period of observation)

            = (6/100,000) × (100)

            = .006

    c. Probability of one case of stomach cancer developing in 100 U.S. person-years?

    $p(x, \mu) = \dfrac{e^{-\mu} \mu^x}{x!}$

        $P = ((e^{-0.006})(.006)^1)/1!$

           $= .994(.006)/1 = .0060$

    d. Number of trials $(n) = 100$

    e. Number of successes $(x) = 1$

    f. Probability of success

            = 6/100,000

            = .00006

    g. Probability of one case of stomach cancer developing in 100 U.S. person-years?

    $P = \binom{N}{x} p^x (1-p)^{N-x}$

    $P(x = 1) = ((100!)/1!) \times (100-1)!)(.00006)^{100}(.99994)^{100-1}$

        $P = .006$

7.

a. $D = 10$ Gy

b. $D_0 = 2$ Gy

c. Surviving fraction $= 1 - (1 - e^{-D/D_0})^n = .0067 = .6\%$

8.

a. 95% confidence interval = 95% CI = Mean +/− (SEM*z)

Mean = 65 years

SEM = standard deviation/n = 9.4/(300) = .54

$z = 1.96$

95% CI = 65 +/− (.54 × 1.96) = 65 +/− 1.06 = 63.94 to 66.06

b. You would expect 19 of these samples to include the population mean.

IMPORTANT STATISTICAL CONCEPTS FOR ONCOLOGISTS

II

Hypothesis Testing

5

In biostatistics, researchers use data to address questions. By convention, the questions are posed as hypotheses, and the data is analyzed to test these hypotheses in a process known as *hypothesis testing*.

In hypothesis testing, we assume that everything occurs by chance (i.e., phenomena are all unrelated to one another and occur independently). Hypothesis testing begins with formation of the *null hypothesis* (H_0), where there is no relationship between two measured phenomena. The null hypothesis is, therefore, often the antithesis of the hypothesis that the researcher is choosing to study.

Example

For example, if an oncologist hypothesizes that a novel agent prolongs overall survival in patients with metastatic cancer who have failed first-line therapy, the null hypothesis (H_0) states, simply, that overall survival would not differ in those receiving the novel agent as compared with those not receiving the novel agent.

To proceed with hypothesis testing, one must assume that the null hypothesis (H_0) is true. If the data is likely to have occurred by chance and not as the result of a relationship between the dependent and independent variables, then the null hypothesis (H_0) is not rejected. If the data is statistically unlikely to have occurred by chance, it is, therefore, likely to have occurred as the result of a relationship between the studied variables, and the null hypothesis (H_0) is rejected.

Getting back to our example: We have our null hypothesis (H_0) that a novel agent is not associated with a change in overall survival in patients with metastatic cancer who have failed-first line therapy. We then collect data from a sample of patients and find that those receiving the novel agent have a median survival that is statistically significantly longer than that of those receiving placebo. The null hypothesis (H_0) is, therefore, rejected.

When the data supports the null hypothesis (H_0), the null hypothesis (H_0) cannot be "accepted;" it can only be "not rejected." Just as observations that contradict a theory serve to disprove it, data that does not support the null hypothesis (H_0) can disprove it. And just as observations that are consistent with a theory cannot prove the theory, data that supports a null hypothesis (H_0) cannot prove it; such data can lead only to not rejecting it.

TYPE I AND TYPE II ERRORS

Statistical conclusions are based on likelihood or chance. With chance comes the potential for error. For hypothesis testing, there are two main types of errors: Type I error and Type II error.

Type I error occurs when the null hypothesis (H_0) is rejected even though it is representative of the truth. In other words, Type I error occurs when the data does not support the null hypothesis although the null hypothesis is true. In the case of Type I error, the data is the result of chance and not of any true relationship between variables being examined. This represents finding evidence of a relationship that does NOT truly exist.

Example

We will use an example of the relationship between the use of a novel agent and risk of developing Grade 3 fatigue. The null hypothesis (H_0) states that there is no relationship between the use of this agent and the risk of Grade 3 fatigue. In an early, small, randomized Phase II trial, 20 patients with metastatic cancer are randomly assigned to receive standard of care versus standard of care plus the addition of a novel agent. As part of the trial, toxicity data, including grade of fatigue, is collected. Analysis of the data collected reveals that, in the subjects studied, the rate of Grade 3 fatigue is higher among patients receiving the novel agent than among those not receiving the novel agent. The null hypothesis (H_0) is rejected based on this data, and the investigators conclude that the use of the agent is associated with increased risk of Grade 3 fatigue. Multiple later Phase III studies with larger sample sizes show no such relationship between use of the novel agent and increase in fatigue of any grade. The finding of the initial Phase II study is likely the result of Type I error.

Type II error occurs when the null hypothesis (H_0) is not rejected despite that it is not representative of the truth. In other words, a Type II error occurs when the data supports a null hypothesis even though the null hypothesis is not true. This represents NOT finding a relationship that, in reality, does exist.

Example

An example of a Type II error is as follows: A small group of 20 patients with metastatic cancer is randomly assigned to receive standard of care or standard of care plus the addition of a novel agent. The null hypothesis (H_0) states that overall survival would not differ in those receiving the novel agent as compared with those receiving the novel agent plus placebo. Overall survival is examined, and it is found that the median survival is the same between those who received the novel agent and those who did not. The null hypothesis is not rejected based on this data, and the investigators conclude that the use of the agent is NOT associated with an improvement in overall survival in patients with metastatic cancer. Multiple studies with larger sample sizes show that patients with metastatic cancer treated with the novel agent have a longer median survival than those not treated with the agent. The negative finding of the initial study likely is the result of Type II error, because the agent does, in fact, improve survival in patients with metastatic cancer.

Another clear way of thinking about Type I and Type II errors is to think of a court room. In a court room, the defendant is innocent until proven guilty. This would mean the null hypothesis (H_0) is that the defendant did not commit the crime. A Type I error is the case in which the defendant is truly innocent, yet the trial results in saying he or she is guilty, sending them to prison. A Type II error is the case in which the defendant truly is guilty but the trial finds him or her innocent. In the court systems and biostatistics, we consider a Type I error to be more important. It is more important to not send an innocent person to prison. In medical terms, we might be testing that a novel treatment is safe. The null hypothesis (H_0) would be that the treatment is not safe. Committing a Type I error would be allowing a dangerous treatment to go into market. The Type II error would be saying that a safe treatment was dangerous.

Alpha and beta are two concepts very important to hypothesis testing. *Alpha* (α) is the level of significance in hypothesis testing determined by the investigator prior to initiation of the experiment as part of the experimental design. Alpha is the probability of rejecting the null hypothesis when it is true. Alpha is, therefore, the probability of making at Type I error. By convention, typical values of alpha specified in medical research are .05 and .01. For the purposes of all examples in this text, we set the alpha value at .05 unless otherwise stated.

Beta (β) is the probability of not rejecting the null hypothesis when it is not true. Beta is, therefore, the probability of making a Type II error. Typical values for beta are .10 to .20. Beta is directly related to the power of a statistical test. *Power* is the probability of correctly rejecting the null hypothesis when it is not true.

$$Power = 1 - Beta.$$

To remember the distinction between Type I and Type II error, think of the relationship between alpha (α) and Type I error and beta (β) and Type II error as being in alphabetical and numeric order:

Alpha, (α) **(A)** is the probability	of making Type I error **(1)**
Beta, (β) **(B)** is the probability	of making Type II error **(2)**

p-VALUES

Decisions in hypothesis testing are based on the likelihood that the data is the result of random chance versus the likelihood that the data is the result of a relationship between the phenomena being investigated. *p*-values are calculated to determine these chances. *p*-values are everywhere in statistics and very often misinterpreted. It is very important that we understand and interpret them correctly.

A *p*-value is a probability; it represents the probability of obtaining the data and results by chance. If we perform a statistical test to test a null hypothesis (H_0), and testing yields a *p*-value of .25, then the probability that the results are due to chance is 25%.

The *p*-value is intricately related to the α level. To minimize the effects of chance on biostatistical conclusions, the α level is set quite low by convention in most biostatistical tests and clinical trials. At an α level of .05, a *p*-value of less than .05 is required to achieve statistical significance. If a statistical test is carried out and a *p*-value less than .05 is calculated, the null hypothesis is rejected. The likelihood that the null hypothesis is rejected based on chance alone is less than 5%.

Recently, the American Statistical Association (ASA) released a statement on statistical significance and *p*-values (1). The following six principles were outlined to guide investigators, researchers, and clinicians in use and interpretation of *p*-values:

- *p*-values can indicate how incompatible the data are with a specified statistical model.
- *p*-values do not measure the probability that the studied hypothesis is true, or the probability that the data was produced by random chance alone.

- Scientific conclusions and business or policy decisions should not be based only on whether a p-value passes a specific threshold.
- Proper inference requires full reporting and transparency.
- A p-value, or statistical significance, does not measure the size of an effect or the importance of a result.
- By itself, a p-value does not provide a good measure of evidence regarding a model or hypothesis.

In many cases, using interval estimates along with the point estimates provides a much clearer understanding of the data than the p-values alone.

t-TESTS

A *t-test* is used to compare the means of two normally distributed samples. It is one of the most basic biostatistics tests.

A *t*-test is useful if we want to test whether there is a difference between two samples based on differences in the means of the two samples. The data analyzed via a *t*-test must be quantitative and continuous. A *t*-test is used most appropriately for samples that are normally distributed.

Example

A breast surgeon knows that triple-negative breast cancer is more likely to affect younger women. She decides to evaluate her patient population to compare the ages of those with triple-negative breast cancer to those with ER+, PR+, and Her2- breast cancers. The surgeon has performed breast surgeries for 293 new breast cancer diagnoses in the past five years. Of these, 52 women had triple-negative breast cancers, and 159 had breast cancers that were ER+, PR+, and Her2-. The average age of the women with TN breast cancer is 53.9 years, and the average age of those with ER+, PR+, and Her2- breast cancer is 60 years. The null hypothesis (H_0) is that there is no difference between the ages of patients in the two samples.

To perform a *t*-test, one must know the mean of each sample, the standard deviation or the standard error of the mean and the number of patients in each sample. The *t*-statistic is calculated using Equation 5.1:

$$t = \frac{\overline{x}_1 - \overline{x}_2}{\sqrt{\frac{s_1^2}{n_1} + \frac{s_2^2}{n_2}}} \tag{5.1}$$

For this example, the breast surgeon collects the following data:

A sample of 20 patients with breast cancer representing the triple-negative population are the following ages (years):

55, 63, 49, 44, 58, 39, 67, 66, 44, 58, 39, 42, 51, 62, 65, 47, 70, 44, 50, 64

Mean age = 53.85

Standard deviation = 10.16

Standard error of the mean = 2.27

A sample of 20 patients with breast cancer representing the ER+, PR+, and Her2- population are the following ages (years):

73, 59, 72, 44, 65, 66, 55, 55, 52, 59, 68, 54, 48, 67, 56, 69, 52, 51, 64, 70

Mean age = 59.95

Standard deviation = 8.57

Standard error of the mean = 1.92

$t = 2.052$

$df = 38$

Standard error of the difference = 2.97

$p = .0471$

The p-value is less than .05 (the predetermined alpha level); therefore, the null hypothesis is rejected, and the breast surgeon concludes that the average age of her patients with triple-negative breast cancer is different than the average age of her patients with ER+, PR+, and Her2- breast cancer.

ONE-TAILED VERSUS TWO-TAILED

The number of tails used in a t-test (one- vs. two-tailed) is dependent upon on the hypothesis and the null hypothesis being tested. If an investigator is hypothesizing that there is a difference between the means of two samples, but the hypothesis does not specify which of those two means will be greater, then a two-tailed t-test is most appropriate. The difference between the two means could be in either direction. A two-tailed t-test is carried out such that the level of significance, α, is divided at each end of the probability distribution.

Example

Using the example examining age and molecular subtype of breast cancer, a two-tailed *t*-test would test the hypothesis that mean age of those with triple-negative breast cancer is different from the mean age of those with ER+, PR+, and Her2- breast cancer. The investigator's hypothesis is nondirectional. The null hypothesis (H_0) would state that there is no difference between the mean ages of the two samples.

So, if the alpha level is set at .05, the two-tailed *t*-test allows that a result would be statistically significant if the likelihood that women with triple-negative breast cancer were significantly younger by random chance was less than 2.5% or if the likelihood that women with triple-negative breast cancer were significantly older by random chance was less than 2.5% as shown in Figure 5.1.

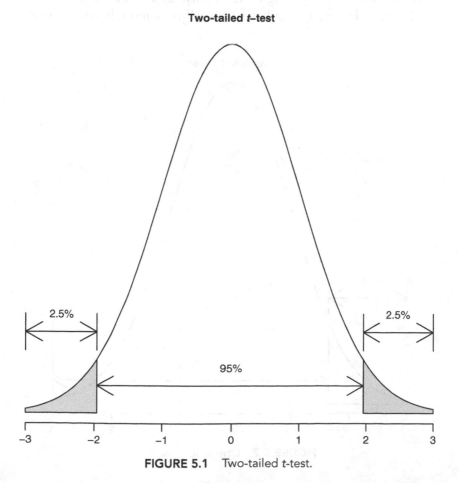

FIGURE 5.1 Two-tailed t-test.

For the same investigation, a one-tailed *t*-test would test the hypothesis that the mean age of those with triple-negative breast cancer is younger than the mean age of those with ER+, PR+, and Her2- breast cancer. The null hypothesis (H_0) would state that the mean age of those with triple-negative breast cancer is not lower than the mean age of those with ER+, PR+, and Her2- breast cancer. So, if the alpha level is set at .05, the one-tailed *t*-test allows that a result would be statistically significant if the likelihood that women with triple-negative breast cancer were significantly younger by random chance was less than 5% as shown in Figure 5.2.

The one-tailed test allows for a higher chance of Type I error. A one-tailed test is generally cautioned against unless there is strong existing evidence to support a directional difference. In the case of this example, there is a great deal of literature to support that triple-negative breast cancers are more common among younger women than among older women.

Seems simple enough, right? In reality, almost all *t*-tests in oncologic biostatistics are two-tailed *t*-tests. This is most likely because a

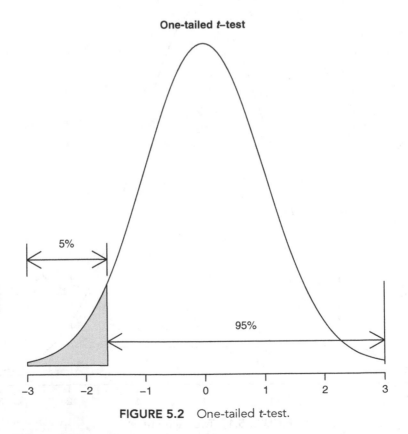

FIGURE 5.2 One-tailed *t*-test.

one-tailed test only accounts for a one-directional scenario, and thereby can lead to inaccurate and biased results; a one tailed test increases the chance for Type I error. So, the example of comparing the average age of women with triple-negative breast cancer versus the average age of women with ER+, PR+, and Her2- breast cancer would most commonly be carried out as a two-tailed *t*-test, despite the existing evidence showing that triple-negative breast cancers are more common among younger women.,

INDEPENDENT SAMPLES

Two samples that contain subjects that are in no way related are considered independent samples. To compare the means of these samples, one would use an *independent t-test*. The preceding example comparing mean ages among groups of women with different biologic subtypes of breast cancer is an example of an independent *t*-test.

PAIRED DATA

In some cases, there is a relationship between the two samples whose means are being compared.

Example

For example, a group of patients may have their blood pressure checked before and after receiving an intervention. The pre- and post-intervention blood pressure would be considered paired data because the data for the pre-intervention group comes from the same patient as the data from the post-intervention group. The pre-treatment blood pressure for each patient is related to and paired with the post-treatment blood pressure for the same patient. A paired *t*-test would be appropriate.

Example

Going back to our example of comparing the average age of women with triple-negative and ER+, PR+, and Her2- breast cancer, obviously we cannot have the same patients in each group. In order to make this study appropriate for a paired *t*-test, we can create a relationship between the two groups, such as matching them for appropriate factors, including tumor, node and metastasis (TNM) stage. With such a matched pair patient sample, a paired *t*-test would be appropriate.

WILCOXON TESTS

WILCOXON RANK-SUM TEST

The Wilcoxon rank-sum test is a nonparametric test similar to the independent t-test used to compare the means of two independent samples that are not normally distributed.

WILCOXON SIGNED-RANK TEST

The Wilcoxon signed-rank test is a nonparametric test similar to the paired t-test used to compare the means of two paired samples that are not normally distributed.

ANALYSIS OF VARIANCE

Comparison of means for more than two groups should not be carried out with multiple t-tests (for normally distributed populations) or multiple Wilcoxon rank-sum tests (for non-normally distributed data). Multiple comparisons using these methods designed to compare two means can lead to issues with increased Type I error due to multiple testing. Thus, such an analysis comparing multiple means should be carried out using an analysis of variance (ANOVA).

Example

The breast surgeon who compared the mean age of women with triple-negative breast cancer to the mean age of women with ER+, PR+, and Her2- breast cancer decides to evaluate her population to compare the ages of her patients in groups based upon the four main molecular phenotypes of breast cancer: Luminal A, Luminal B, Her2-enriched, and Basal-like. The surgeon has performed breast surgeries for 293 new breast cancer diagnoses in the past five years. On extensive pathologic testing, 50 of these 293 women had Basal-like breast cancer, 165 had Luminal A type breast cancer, 43 had Luminal B type breast cancer, and 35 had Her2-enriched breast cancer. The average age of the women with Basal-like breast cancer is 52 years (standard deviation = 10 years); the average age of those with Luminal A type breast cancer is 61 years (standard deviation = 8.5 years); the average age of those with Luminal B type breast cancer is 60 years (standard deviation = 9 years); and the average age of those with Her2-enriched breast cancer is 58 years (standard deviation = 9.5 years).

The null hypothesis (H_0) states that there is no difference between the ages of patients in these four samples. The appropriate statistical test to test this null hypothesis is ANOVA.

ANOVA is a computationally robust comparison of multiple means that is often carried out with a statistical calculator. For the preceding example, ANOVA calculation for the means of these four groups would give a sum of squares between groups and within groups, degrees of freedom between groups and within groups, variance between groups and within groups, an F statistic, and a p-value as shown in the following table:

	Sum of Squares	Degrees of Freedom	Variance	F	p
Between groups	3187.5	3	1062.5	13.2	.0000
Within groups	23219.5	289	80.3		

Based on this calculation and the p-value of less than .00001, we would reject the null hypothesis and conclude that there is a statistically significant difference between the ages of patients in these four groups. Note: even though the p-value states .0000 in the output, it is never truly 0, it just rounds that way to four decimal places. We then say the p-value is less than .00001.

Post-hoc analyses may also be carried out comparing each group to the others, for example, comparing those with Basal-like breast cancer to those with Luminal A breast cancer, comparing those with Basal-like breast cancer to those with Luminal B breast cancer, and comparing those with Basal-like breast cancer to those with Her2-enriched breast cancer. These analyses are not testing a pre-specified hypothesis and are meant to be hypothesis generating.

TESTING BINOMIAL PROPORTIONS

A test of binomial proportions is used to compare proportions among subjects in different groups. A randomized clinical trial looking at relative proportions of side effects between experimental groups is an excellent example of testing binomial proportions.

Example

For many years, axillary lymph node dissection was the standard of care for all patients with breast cancer. This was until three large multicenter trials randomized women with clinically node-negative breast cancer with negative sentinel lymph nodes (SLN) on sentinel lymph node biopsy (SLNB) to axillary lymph node dissection (ALND) or no further axillary surgery. In each of these trials the proportion of patients with complications, particularly lymphedema, was compared between the two groups.

For such a comparison, the null hypothesis (H_0) states that there is no difference in the proportion of patients developing lymphedema in the ALND versus in the axillary SLNB groups. In one of the well-known randomized trials, a total of 3,986 women with negative SLNs were randomly assigned in the study: 1,975 to ALND following SLNB and 2,011 to no further surgery following SLNB. Data regarding lymphedema was available on 1,975 node-negative women randomly assigned to the ALND group and 2,008 node-negative women assigned to the no further surgery following SLNB group. Rates of lymphedema, measured as arm difference greater than 10% at 36 months were compared between the two groups. About 14% of the women in the ALND group and 8% of women in the SLNB group were found to have lymphedema. The difference in lymphedema incidence between the two groups was statistically significant with a p-value of less than .01 (2).

CONFIDENCE INTERVALS AND HYPOTHESIS TESTS: HOW ARE THEY RELATED?

Remember the discussion of confidence intervals in the section titled Interval Estimates, located in Chapter 4? A confidence interval (CI) is a range of values used to estimate an unknown parameter. A CI is often used to estimate a population mean using sample means. But, how does that relate to hypothesis testing?

The CI is equal to $1 - \alpha$. An example of a 95% CI in hypothesis testing can be easily illustrated using a t-test.

Example

It will perhaps be simplest to use the preceding two-tailed t-test example:

A breast surgeon evaluates her patient population to compare the ages of those with triple-negative breast cancer to those with ER+, PR+, and Her2- breast cancer. Among the women on whom she has performed surgery over the past five years, 52 women had triple-negative breast cancers and 159 had breast cancers that were ER+, PR+, and Her2-. The average age of the women with triple-negative breast cancer is 53.9 years and the average age of those with ER+, PR+, and Her2- breast cancer is 60 years. The null hypothesis (H$_0$) states that there is no difference between the mean ages of the two samples. The alternative hypothesis would be that mean age of those with triple-negative breast cancer is different from the mean age of those with ER+, PR+, and Her2- breast cancer.

In the case of this example, α is set at .05. The CI is, therefore, 1 – .05 = .95. So, for this example, as discussed, we focus on the 95% CI.

Using the previously analyzed data samples:

A sample of 20 patients with breast cancer representing the triple-negative population are the following ages (years):

55, 63, 49, 44, 58, 39, 67, 66, 44, 58, 39, 42, 51, 62, 65, 47, 70, 44, 50, 64

Mean age = 53.85

Standard deviation = 10.16

Standard error of the mean = 2.27

A sample of 20 patients with breast cancer representing the ER+, PR+, and Her 2- population are the following ages (years):

73, 59, 72, 44, 65, 66, 55, 55, 52, 59, 68, 54, 48, 67, 56, 69, 52, 51, 64, 70

Mean age = 59.95

Standard deviation = 8.57

Standard error of the mean = 1.92

To calculate the 95% CI (which corresponds to an α of .05), we start by calculating the difference between the two means. Here, the difference between the two means (59.95 – 53.85) is 6.1. The standard error of the difference is calculated by Equation 5.2:

$$\text{Standard error of the difference} = \sqrt{\frac{\sigma_1^2}{n_1} + \frac{\sigma_2^2}{n_2}} \qquad (5.2)$$

For this example, the standard error of the difference would be calculated as follows:

$$\sqrt{\frac{\sigma_1^2}{n_1} + \frac{\sigma_2^2}{n_2}} = \sqrt{\frac{10.16^2}{20} + \frac{8.57^2}{20}} = \sqrt{5.16 + 3.67} = 2.97$$

The standard error of the difference of the means is 2.97

As detailed in the section, Interval Estimates, located in Chapter 4, to calculate the 95% CI, we use Equation 5.3:

$$CI = \bar{x} \pm z^* \frac{\sigma}{\sqrt{n}}. \qquad (5.3)$$

For the 95% CI, we substitute $z = 1.96$. Based on this formula, the 95% CI would be:

$$95\% \text{ CI} = 6.1 \pm 1.96 \times 2.97$$

$$= 6.1 \pm 5.8212$$

$$= (.2788, 11.9212).$$

Because this CI does not include 0, the results are statistically significant.

Looking at this a different way, from the perspective of the alpha level and p-value, the calculated t-statistic is 2.052 and the corresponding two tailed p-value is .0471. The p-value is less than the alpha level, so the null hypothesis is rejected and the results are statistically significant.

What if we use a 99% CI and an alpha level of .01? The difference between the two means remains 6.1 and the standard error of the difference remains 2.97. To calculate the 99% CI, we roughly use the formula:

$$CI = \bar{x} \pm z^* \frac{\sigma}{\sqrt{n}}.$$

For the 99% CI, we substitute $z = 2.58$. Based on this formula, the 99% CI would be:

$$99\% \text{ CI} = 6.1 \pm 2.58 \times 2.97$$

$$= 6.1 \pm 7.6626$$

$$= (-1.5626, 13.7626).$$

Because this CI includes 0, the results are not statistically significant.

Looking at this a different way, from the perspective of the alpha level and p-value, the calculated t-statistic remains 2.052 and the corresponding two tailed p-value is .0471. The p-value is greater than the alpha level (.01), so the null hypothesis is not rejected and the results are statistically significant.

CIs are also helpful to estimate the size of an effect. Remember that the ASA statement on p-values clearly states that a p-value does not measure the size of an effect or the importance of a result (1). A CI is the most appropriate way to estimate effect size (although a CI is not an absolute measure of effect size). An investigator can conclude that, if a study or clinical trials were repeated an infinite number of times and a 95% CI were calculated for each of those, 95% of those CIs would include the true effect size.

SENSITIVITY AND SPECIFICITY

The concepts of sensitivity and specificity are critical to the evaluation of medical, in particular oncologic, diagnostic tests.

Sensitivity is the proportion of patients with a disease who test positive. *Specificity* is the proportion of patients without the disease who test negative. Thus, for a test that is very *sensitive*, a negative test means that there is a high likelihood that the patient does not have the disease. For a test that is very *specific*, a positive test means that there is a high likelihood that the patient actually has the disease.

For any given test, to calculate the numerical value of the sensitivity and specificity, one starts by constructing a 2 × 2 table of the test results (positive versus negative) and the disease status (positive versus negative).

	Presence of disease		
	Positive	Negative	Total
Test result	a	b	$a + b$
Positive			
Negative	c	d	$c + d$
Total	$a + c$	$b + d$	$a + b + c + d$

The formulas for sensitivity (Equation 5.4) and specificity (Equation 5.5) and the related concepts, positive predictive value (Equation 5.6), negative predictive value (Equation 5.7), positive likelihood ratio (Equation 5.8), and negative likelihood ratio (Equation 5.9) are as follows:

True positives = a

False positives = b

True negatives = c

False negatives = d

$$\text{Sensitivity} = \frac{a}{a+c} \qquad (5.4)$$

$$\text{Specificity} = \frac{d}{b+d} \qquad (5.5)$$

Note that to calculate sensitivity and specificity, the denominator is the presence or absence of the disease.

$$\text{Positive Predictive Value (PPV)} = \frac{a}{a+b} \qquad (5.6)$$

$$\text{Negative Predictive Value (NPV)} = \frac{d}{c+d} \qquad (5.7)$$

Note that to calculate NPV and PPV, the denominator is the result of the test.

$$\text{Positive Likelihood Ratio} = \frac{\text{Sensitivity}}{1\text{-Specificity}} \qquad (5.8)$$

$$\text{Negative Likelihood Ratio} = \frac{1\text{-Sensitivity}}{\text{Specificity}} \qquad (5.9)$$

Example

To illustrate the concepts of sensitivity and specificity, we look closely at the example of breast imaging screening studies and their use in women with familial breast cancer (3). The cited study took women with documented BRCA mutations or a greater than 20% lifetime risk of breast cancer, and offered them screening with mammography, ultrasound, and MRI every 12 months at the Medical University of Vienna. A total of 1,365 MRIs, 1,365 mammograms, and 1,365 ultrasounds were performed. In a group of 559 women, 40 cancers were diagnosed. Of these, 36 were detected by MRI, 15 were detected by mammography, and 15 were detected by ultrasound. On MRI, in addition to the 36 cancers, there were an additional 147 suspicious findings that were ultimately found not to be cancers. On mammography there were 38 suspicious findings that were ultimately found not to be cancers, and on ultrasound there were 41 suspicious findings that were ultimately found not to be cancers.

To organize data for this study, 2 × 2 tables would be constructed as follows:

	Presence of breast cancer		
	Positive	Negative	Total
MRI Test result	a	b	
Positive	36	147	183
	c	d	
Negative	4	1,178	1,182
Total	40	1,325	1,365

	Presence of breast cancer		
	Positive	Negative	Total
Ultrasound test result	a	b	
Positive	15	41	56
	c	d	
Negative	25	1,284	1,309
Total	40	1,325	1,365

	Presence of breast cancer		
	Positive	Negative	Total
Mam Test result	a	b	
Positive	15	38	53
	c	d	
Negative	25	1,287	1,312
Total	40	1,325	1,365

Those in box *a* for each test are considered *true positives*—these patients have the disease and appropriately test positive for the disease.

Those in box *b* for each test are referred to as *false positives*—these patients do not have the disease, but do have a positive test.

Those in box *c* are referred to as *false negatives*—these patients have the disease, but have a negative test despite actually having the disease.

Those in box *d* are considered *true negatives*—these patients do not have the disease and appropriately test negative for the disease.

For MRI—The number of patients with the disease who had a positive test was 36. Sensitivity = the number of patients with the disease who had a positive test/the total number of patients with the disease = 36/40 = 90%.

The number of patients without the disease with a negative test was 1,178. Specificity = the number of patients without the disease who had a negative test/the total number of patients without the disease = 1,178/1,325 = 89%

For Mammography—The number of patients with the disease who had a positive test was 15. Sensitivity = the number of patients with the disease who had a positive test divided by the total number of patients with the disease = 15/40 = 37.5%

The number of patients without the disease with a negative test was 1,284. Specificity = the number of patients without the disease who had a negative test/the total number patients without the disease = 1,287/1,325 = 97%

For Ultrasound—The number of patients with the disease who had a positive test was 15. Sensitivity = the number of patients with the disease who had a positive test divided by the total number of patients with the disease = 15/40 = 37.5%

The number of patients without the disease with a negative test was 1,287. Specificity = the number of patients without the disease who had a negative test/the number of patients without the disease = 1,284/1,325 = 97%

REMEMBER: To calculate sensitivity and specificity, the denominator is the presence or absence of the disease!

A comparative review of these tests suggests that MRI is the most sensitive, and mammography and ultrasound are equally specific. Both mammography and ultrasound are more specific than MRI.

Sensitive tests rule out and specific tests rule in. That is to say, if you have a sensitive test, and you get a negative result, then it is very likely that the patient does not have the disease. This is considered the SnOut rule. And, if you have a specific test, and you get a positive result, then it is very likely that the patient does have the disease. This is considered the SpIn rule.

The SpIn and SnOut rules may be best illustrated by calculating the negative predictive value and the positive predictive value.

NEGATIVE PREDICTIVE VALUE

Example

If a patient with a BRCA mutation or greater than 20% lifetime risk of breast cancer has a negative MRI, then there is a 99.7% chance that they do not have the disease. This figure is determined by calculating the negative predictive value. The *negative predictive value* is calculated by taking the number of patients without the disease who have a negative test and dividing that by the number of patients with a negative test = 1,178/1,182 = 99.7%. Compare that to the negative predictive value of mammography for which 1,287 patients without the disease had a negative test, and for which a total of 1,312 patients had a negative test = 1,287/1,312 = 98%. With the more sensitive test (MRI), a negative test is more likely to rule out the disease—hence, the SnOut rule.

POSITIVE PREDICTIVE VALUE

Mammography is more specific than MRI. A positive mammogram is more likely than a positive MRI to be associated with a cancer diagnosis. To illustrate the SpIn rule, for each test, we look at the positive predictive value or the number of patients with the disease with a positive test divided by the total number of positive tests. The *positive predictive value* is calculated by taking the number of patients with the disease who have a positive test and dividing that by the number of patients with a positive test. For MRI, the positive predictive value is 36/183 = 19.7%. For mammography, the positive predictive value is 15/53 = 28.3%. A positive mammogram is more likely to rule in the disease than a positive MRI because the mammography is a more specific test—hence, the SpIn rule.

REMEMBER: To calculate NPV and PPV, the denominator is the result of the test!

When considering a diagnostic test, a likelihood ratio helps to estimate the value of performing the test.

POSITIVE LIKELIHOOD RATIO

The positive likelihood ratio is a likelihood ratio for a positive test (i.e., the chance that a positive test will represent a true positive). A likelihood ratio of greater than 1 indicates that the positive test result is likely to be associated with a patient who truly has the disease (a true positive).

The formula for the positive likelihood ratios is: $\dfrac{\text{sensitivity}}{(1-\text{specificity})}$.

In other words, the positive likelihood ratio is calculated from the probability of a person who has the disease testing positive divided by the probability of a person who does not have the disease testing positive.

So, for MRI in the preceding example, the positive likelihood ratio is $\dfrac{.9}{(1-.89)} = \dfrac{.9}{.11} = 8.1$. Based on this result, a positive MRI has a moderate effect on increasing the probability of breast cancer.

NEGATIVE LIKELIHOOD RATIO

The negative likelihood ratio is a likelihood ratio for a negative test (i.e., the chance that a negative test will represent a true negative). A negative likelihood ratio of greater than 1 indicates that the test result is likely to be associated with a patient who does not truly have the disease (a true negative).

The formula for the negative likelihood ratios is : $\dfrac{1-\text{sensitivity}}{\text{specificity}}$.

In other words, the negative likelihood ratio is calculated from the probability of a person who has the disease testing negative divided by the probability of a person who does not have the disease testing negative.

For MRI, in the preceding example, the positive likelihood ratio is $\dfrac{(1-.9)}{.89} = \dfrac{.1}{.89} = .11$. Based on this result, a negative MRI has a moderate to large effect on decreasing the probability of breast cancer.

REFERENCES

1. Wasserstein RL, Lazar NA. The ASA's statement on *p*-values: context, process, and purpose. *Am Stat.* 2016;70:129–133. doi:10.1080/0003130 5.2016.1154108
2. Ashikga T, Krag DN, Land SR, et al. Morbidity results from the NSABP B-32 trial comparing sentinel lymph node dissection vs. axillary dissection. *J Surg Oncol.* 2010;102:111–118. doi:10.1002/jso.21535
3. Riedl CC, Luft N, Bernhart C, et al. Triple-modality screening trial of familial breast cancer underlines the importance of magnetic resonance imaging and questions the role of mammography and ultrasound regardless of patient mutation status, age, and breast density. *J Clin Oncol.* 2015;33:1128–1135. doi:10.1200/JCO.2014.56.8626

Correlation and Regression 6

We use both correlation and regression to discuss relationships between variables.

CORRELATION

A *correlation* examines the linear relationship between two quantitative variables. This is often thought of as a way to investigate a relationship between two independent variables. A *correlation coefficient* measures the extent to which two variables tend to change together. The coefficient describes both the strength and the direction of the relationship.

PEARSON CORRELATION COEFFICIENT

Pearson product moment correlation coefficient, which is the most commonly taught correlation coefficient, is strongly biased toward linear trends.

Example

Let us use the example of the correlation between tumor diameter and number of involved lymph nodes in breast cancer. We use a fictional example data set of 24 patients with breast cancer who have undergone breast and axillary surgery. The diameter of the primary tumor and number of axillary lymph nodes are presented in table form in the following text:

Tumor Diameter (cm)	Number of Axillary Lymph Nodes Involved
2.1	1
1.1	0
.5	0

(continued)

Tumor Diameter (cm)	Number of Axillary Lymph Nodes Involved
1.7	2
5.5	15
3.4	3
.8	0
1.3	1
.4	0
2.1	0
1.0	0
1.8	0
2.8	2
.8	0
1.1	0
1.8	0
2.2	2
1.9	1
1.3	0
.9	0
3.2	1
4.8	5
1.5	0
1.2	0

Graphically, a correlation can be displayed as a scatter plot (Figure 6.1).

The first goal of a Pearson product moment correlation test is to determine if there exists a linear relationship between two variables. As with most biostatistical tests, tests of correlation lend themselves to hypothesis testing. For our example, the null hypothesis (H_0) would be that there is no linear relationship between tumor diameter and risk of involved axillary lymph nodes. Both tumor diameter and number of involved lymph nodes are considered independent variables.

A correlation coefficient calculator is used to calculate the correlation coefficient, and then a p-value is obtained using the correlation coefficient and sample size, n. In the case of our example, the correlation coefficient

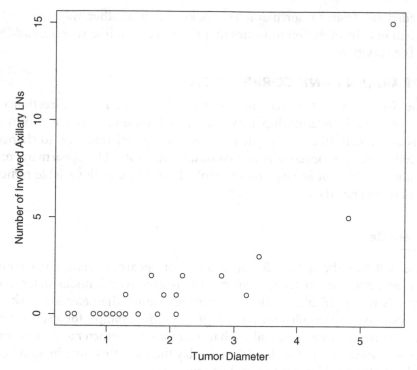

FIGURE 6.1 Scatter plot of the relationship between tumor diameter and number of involved axillary lymph nodes (LNs).

$r = .82459$, $n = 24$, and the p-value is less than .001. Based upon this p-value, we reject the null hypothesis, and conclude that a linear relationship does exist between tumor diameter and number of involved axillary lymph nodes.

The second goal of a correlation is to describe how tightly the two variables are associated. This is usually expressed with the correlation coefficient r, which ranges from -1 to 1, or the coefficient of determination r^2, which ranges from 0 to 1.

For this example, the correlation coefficient $r = .82459$ and the coefficient of determination $r^2 = .67995$. This is considered a positive correlation, because r has a positive value indicating that as the tumor diameter increases, so does the number of involved lymph nodes. A negative correlation would describe the opposite linear relationship; as the X variable goes up, the Y variable goes down.

The coefficient of determination r^2 represents the extent to which one variable is predictable from the other variable. In the case of this example, 68% of the variance of the number of involved lymph nodes is predictable from tumor diameter. Looking at it another way, the coefficient of determination indicates that the regression line represents 68% of the variation.

SPEARMAN RANK CORRELATION

The *Spearman rank correlation* measures the strength and direction of the monotonic relationship between ranked variables (either continuous or ordinal). In a monotonic relationship, the variables tend to change together, but not necessarily at a constant linear rate. The Spearman correlation coefficient is based on the ranked values for each variable rather than on the raw data.

Example

The null hypothesis (H_0) for an analysis of Spearman rank correlation between tumor diameter and number of involved lymph nodes states that there is no significant relationship between tumor diameter and risk of involved axillary lymph nodes. To adapt the earlier example for a Spearman rank correlation, we must rank both the tumor size/diameter and the number of involved lymph nodes. We redisplay the data, this time in a ranked order. Both variables must be ranked separately.

Tumor Size (cm)	Tumor Size Rank	Number of Involved Lymph Nodes (LNs)	Number of Involved LN Rank
.4	1	0	7.5
.5	2	0	7.5
.8	3	0	7.5
.8	4	0	7.5
.9	5	0	7.5
1	6	0	7.5
1.1	7.5	0	7.5
1.1	7.5	0	7.5
1.2	9	0	7.5
1.3	10.5	1	17
1.3	10.5	0	7.5
1.5	12	0	7.5

(continued)

Tumor Size (cm)	Tumor Size Rank	Number of Involved Lymph Nodes (LNs)	Number of Involved LN Rank
1.7	13	1	17
1.8	14.5	0	7.5
1.8	14.5	0	7.5
1.9	16	1	17
2.1	17.5	1	17
2.1	17.5	0	7.5
2.2	19	1	17
2.8	20	2	20.5
3.2	21	2	20.5
3.4	22	3	22
4.8	23	5	23
5.5	24	15	24

When identical values exist in the data (in either variable), one must take the average of the ranks that they would have otherwise occupied. The most complicated example of this, shown in the previous table, is that there are 14 values of "0" for involved lymph nodes. To create the rank of these 14 values, one must perform the following calculation:

$$((1+2+3+4+5+6+7+8+9+10+11+12+13+14)/14)) = 105/14 = 7.5$$

So each of these 14 values of "0" receives a rank of 7.5. This is because there is no way to distinguish which of the "0" values should be ranked number 1, which should be ranked number 14, and which ones should be ranked in between.

The next step is to calculate the Spearman's Rho correlation coefficient R. This is a multistep process best performed by the Spearman's Rho calculator.

Spearman's correlation coefficient R = .8079, This R corresponds to a p-value of .000002. Based on this p-value, we reject the null hypothesis and conclude that there is a significant relationship between tumor diameter and risk of involved axillary lymph nodes.

REGRESSION

Medical researchers most often use regression as a summary of data. When considering the hypothesis tests and correlations, we were limited in how many variables we could compare to one another. With *t*-tests and analysis of variance (ANOVA), we were comparing means of one variable being grouped by another; with correlation, we were comparing only two variables to each other. Such tests are very limiting considering most medical studies desire to adjust for age, sex, and race (at a minimum) in addition to many other characteristics. This is where regression comes in. With regression, we mathematically relate one variable to one or more other variables.

SIMPLE LINEAR REGRESSION

With a *simple linear regression*, scores from one independent variable are used to predict scores on a dependent continuous variable.

Example

Carrying over the earlier example, we define the independent variable as tumor diameter and the dependent variable as number of involved axillary lymph nodes.

INDEPENDENT VARIABLE Tumor Diameter (cm)	DEPENDENT VARIABLE Number of Axillary Lymph Nodes Involved
2.1	1
1.1	0
.5	0
1.7	2
5.5	15
3.4	3
.8	0
1.3	1
.4	0
2.1	0
1.0	0
1.8	0
2.8	2
.8	0

(continued)

| INDEPENDENT VARIABLE | DEPENDENT VARIABLE |
Tumor Diameter (cm)	Number of Axillary Lymph Nodes Involved
1.1	0
1.8	0
2.2	2
1.9	1
1.3	0
.9	0
3.2	1
4.8	5
1.5	0
1.2	0

Graphically, a regression is displayed as a scatter plot with a best-fit line (Figure 6.2).

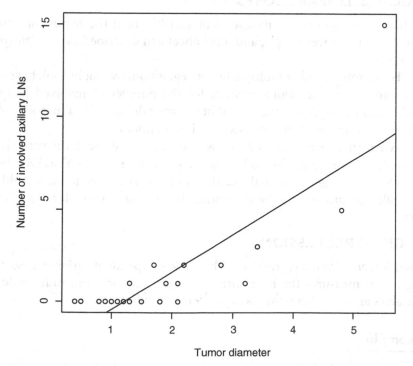

FIGURE 6.2   Linear regression with best-fit line for tumor diameter and number of involved axillary lymph nodes.

A best-fit line is developed with the equation $y = mx + b$ where m is the slope of the line and b is the y intercept. We can estimate the linear regression equation for the earlier data set:

The slope (m) is roughly 2/1 (you rise 2 units on the y-axis for every 1 unit on the x-axis) and the y-intercept is roughly -2.5. Thus, the regression equation can be estimated at $y = 2x - 2.5$. This equation can be used to predict the number of positive lymph nodes for a given tumor diameter.

What would be the predicted number of lymph nodes positive for a 5-cm tumor?

Using the best-fit line equation, we calculate: $y = 2^*(x) - 2.5 = 7.5$

By calculation and by looking at the best-fit line, we would predict seven to eight positive lymph nodes if the primary tumor measures 5 cm.

The decision of which variable you call "X" and which you call "Y" matters in regression, as you will get a different best-fit line if you swap the two. The line that best predicts Y from X is not the same as the line that predicts X from Y. The X is typically the independent variable and the Y is the dependent variable.

MULTIPLE LINEAR REGRESSION

If there is more than one independent variable, then the regression relationship is no longer simple, and it is henceforth described as *multiple linear regression*.

For example, with a multiple linear regression, we might look beyond how tumor diameter alone predicts for the number of involved lymph nodes, and we might instead look at how tumor diameter and tumor grade predict for number of involved axillary lymph nodes.

When there are both continuous and categorical predictor variables, multiple regression is also called *analysis of covariance (ANCOVA)*. For an ANCOVA regression analysis, the continuous independent variables are called *covariates* and the categorical independent variables are called *factors*.

LOGISTIC REGRESSION

Logistic regression is a regression with a binary dependent variable. Logistic regression measures the relationship between one or more independent variables and the dichotomous dependent variable.

Example

It may be particularly illustrative to continue with the same example used for correlation and linear regression—in this case, the dependent variable should be a categorical binary/dichotomous variable. To adapt the previous example, the independent variable remains a continuous variable of tumor diameter and our dependent variable is a dichotomous nominal variable—negative lymph nodes (no positive lymph nodes) versus positive lymph nodes. The data would be collected as follows:

Tumor Diameter (cm)	Lymph Node Status (Negative vs. Positive/yes vs. no)
.4	Negative/no
.5	Negative/no
.8	Negative/no
.8	Negative/no
.9	Negative/no
1	Negative/no
1.1	Negative/no
1.1	Negative/no
1.2	Negative/no
1.3	Positive/yes
1.3	Negative/no
1.5	Negative/no
1.7	Positive/yes
1.8	Negative/no
1.8	Negative/no
1.9	Positive/yes
2.1	Positive/yes
2.1	Negative/no
2.2	Positive/yes
2.8	Positive/yes
3.2	Positive/yes
3.4	Positive/yes
4.8	Positive/yes
5.5	Positive/yes

The goal of analysis using a logistic regression is to estimate conditional probabilities, meaning that we are able to predict the likelihood that a woman with breast cancer will have positive lymph nodes based on the diameter of the tumor. The statistical null hypothesis (H_0) is that the probability of positive lymph nodes is not associated with the tumor diameter; in other words, the line describing the relationship between the tumor diameter and the probability of positive lymph nodes has a slope of zero.

The difference between linear and logistic regression is that logistic regression does not measure the dependent variable directly; it instead estimates the probability of yes versus no in a dichotomous variable. Output of a logistic regression calculator is shown in the following text:

PREDICTED PROBABILITY OF OUTCOME, WITH 95% CONFIDENCE LIMITS

X	Y	Probability	Low	High
.4000	0	.0066	.0001	.2994
.5000	0	.0093	.0002	.3127
.8000	0	.0263	.0013	.3588
.8000	0	.0263	.0013	.3588
.9000	0	.0369	.0024	.3769
1.0000	0	.0517	.0045	.3972
1.1000	0	.0719	.0082	.4201
1.1000	0	.0719	.0082	.4201
1.2000	0	.0991	.0148	.4468
1.3000	1	.1352	.0260	.4784
1.3000	0	.1352	.0260	.4784
1.5000	0	.2399	.0713	.5650
1.7000	1	.3893	.1519	.6940
1.8000	0	.4752	.1978	.7689
1.8000	0	.4752	.1978	.7689
1.9000	1	.5627	.2409	.8392
2.1000	1	.7221	.3118	.9371
2.1000	0	.7221	.3118	.9371
2.2000	1	.7869	.3404	.9635
2.8000	1	.9681	.4631	.9991
3.2000	1	.9920	.5253	.9999

(continued)

X	Y	Probability	Low	High
3.4000	1	.9960	.5537	1.0000
4.8000	1	1.0000	.7203	1.0000
5.5000	1	1.0000	.7846	1.0000

Overall model fit

Chi square = 17.5366

Degrees of freedom = 1

$p = .0000$

Based on the p-value of less than .00001, we reject the null hypothesis.

This is an example of a simple logistic regression with a single independent variable and a dichotomous dependent variable. A multiple logistic regression would be appropriate to analyze the relationship between more than one independent variable and a categorical dependent variable.

Categorical Data Analysis

Often, all variables to be analyzed are categorical.

CONTINGENCY TABLES

2 × 2 TABLES

A 2 × 2 contingency table is an excellent way to organize two dichotomous categorical variables. The table displays the frequency of two values of two variables.

Example

Let us use a fictional example dataset of 1,026 patients with metastatic lung cancer. We are given Karnofsky performance status (KPS) as less than 70 or greater than or equal to 70, and information about whether the patients have brain metastases or no brain metastases (extracranial disease only).

In this population, 406 patients (40% of patients) have a KPS less than 70 and 620 patients (60% of patients) have a KPS greater than or equal to 70. In total, 442 patients (43% of patients) have no brain metastases/ extracranial disease only, and 584 patients (57% of patients) have brain metastases.

A 2 × 2 contingency table would look like this:

	No Brain Metastases/ Extracranial Disease Only	Brain Metastases	Total
KPS <70	104	302	406
KPS ≥70	338	282	620
Total	442	584	1026

R × C TABLES

R × C contingency tables are also known as row × column contingency tables. *R × C contingency tables* are appropriate to organize and display multiple variables that are categorical but not necessarily dichotomous.

Example

An example of such an R × C contingency table can be found in a recent publication examining associations between clinicopathologic features and mismatch repair (MMR) defects in endometroid endometrial cancer (EEC) in an NRG Oncology/Gynecologic Oncology Group study (1).

		MMR Normal	Epigenetic MMR Defect	Probable MMR Mutation	MSI Low
Age	<60	311	82	63	7
	≥60	328	182	36	15
BMI	<25	72	37	26	2
	≥25–30	121	48	23	6
	≥30–35	135	78	15	5
	≥35	309	100	35	9
Race	White	572	243	92	19
	Black	38	14	5	1
	Other	29	7	2	2
Grade	1	295	89	38	9
	2	260	132	37	11
	3	84	43	24	2
Stage	I	491	181	81	18
	II	63	25	5	1
	III	72	57	9	3
	IV	13	1	4	0
LVI	+	108	87	30	3
	–	518	173	67	19

(*continued*)

		MMR Normal	Epigenetic MMR Defect	Probable MMR Mutation	MSI Low
Depth of invasion	None	119	30	19	3
	Inner half	344	151	50	12
	Outer half and serosal	160	76	24	7
Adjuvant therapy	Any adjuvant therapy	111	63	26	5
	No further treatment	526	200	73	17

FISHER'S EXACT TEST

Fisher's exact test is one way to test associations between data in contingency tables. This test gives an exact p-value (as opposed to an estimate of a p-value).

For a given 2 × 2 contingency table:

	Column 1	Column 2	Total
Row 1	a	b	a + b
Row 2	c	d	c + d
Total	a + c	b + d	a + b + c + d

The p-value for Fisher's exact test is calculated by Equation 7.1:

$$p = \frac{\binom{a+b}{a}\binom{c+d}{c}}{\binom{n}{a+c}} = \frac{(a+b)!(c+d)!(a+c)!(b+d)!}{a!b!c!d!} \qquad (7.1)$$

In many texts, you will read that Fisher's exact test is most appropriately used when the expected values (row total × column total) are relatively small, as this gives a more accurate estimate via an exact p-value. It is often suggested that a rule of thumb is to use Fisher's exact test when the total sample size is less than 1,000. However, many studies have shown that the chi-square test is actually very robust to small cell sizes, as well as small sample sizes (2).

Example

Using the preceding example of patients with metastatic lung cancer, we calculate Fisher's exact test using a Fisher's exact test calculator. The null hypothesis (H_0) for this analysis states that, for patients with metastatic lung cancer, KPS and the presence or absence of brain metastases are independent of one another.

We start with the 2 × 2 contingency table:

	No Brain Metastases/ Extracranial Disease Only	Brain Metastases	Total
KPS <70	104	302	406
KPS ≥70	338	282	620
Total	442	584	1,026

Fisher's exact test calculation reveals a *p*-value of .001. Based on this *p*-value, we reject the null hypothesis, and conclude that there is a relationship between KPS and the presence or absence of brain metastases.

CHI-SQUARE TEST

The *chi-square test* is the most commonly used measurement of association of the data found in contingency tables. The test is formally known as the Pearson's chi-square test, and is designed to determine whether there is a relationship between the row values and the column values. This test gives an estimate of the *p*-value (as opposed to the exact *p*-value given by Fisher's exact test).

Example

Using the example of the 2 × 2 table (KPS × brain metastases), we can go through the steps used to calculate the chi-square test statistic and to test the null hypothesis (H_0).

For this example, the null hypothesis (H_0) states that, for patients with metastatic lung cancer, KPS and the presence or absence of brain metastases are independent of one another.

The steps to calculate the chi-square test are as follows:

Chi-square step 1: Start with 2 × 2 contingency table.

	No Brain Metastases/ Extracranial Disease Only	Brain Metastases	Total
KPS <70	104	302	406
KPS ≥70	338	282	620
Total	442	584	1,026

Chi-square step 2: Calculate the expected values for each cell by the formula:

Expected cell frequency = (Row Total × Column Total)/n, where n = total sample size

	No Brain Metastases/ Extracranial Disease Only	Brain Metastases	Total
KPS <70	104 (406 × 442)/1,026 = 175	302 (406 × 584)/1,026 = 231	406
KPS ≥70	338 (620 × 442)/1,026 = 267	282 (620 × 584)/1,026 = 353	620
Total	442	584	1,026

Chi-square step 3: Calculate the difference between the expected and observed cell frequency.

	No Brain Metastases/ Extracranial Disease Only	Brain Metastases	Total
KPS <70	104 (406 × 442)/1,026 = 175 104–175 = −71	302 (406 × 584)/1,026 = 231 302–231 = 71	406
KPS ≥70	338 (620 × 442)/1,026 = 267 338–267 = 71	282 (620 × 584)/1,026 = 353 282–353 = −71	620
Total	442	584	1,026

Chi-square step 4: Square the calculated difference and then divide by the expected cell frequency.

	Extracranial Disease Only	Brain Metastases	Total
KPS <70	104	302	406
	(406 × 442)/1,026 = 175	(406 × 584)/1,026 = 231	
	104–175 = –71	302–231 = 71	
	$(-71)^2/175 = 29$	$(-71)^2/231 = 22$	
KPS ≥70	338 (620 × 442)/1,026 = 267	282 (620 × 584)/1,026 = 353	620
	338–267 = 71	282–353 = –71	
	$(-71)^2/267 = 19$	$(-71)^2/353 = 14$	
Total	442	584	1,026

Chi-square step 5: The chi-square statistic is computed by summing the last row in each cell.

Chi-square statistic = 29 + 22 + 19 + 14 = 84

Chi-square step 6: Calculate degrees of freedom (df).

Degrees of freedom = (number of rows – 1) × (number of columns – 1) = $1 \times 1 = 1$

Chi-square step 7: The chi-square statistic with associated degrees of freedom corresponds to an estimated *p*-value. In this case, the estimated *p*-value is less than .0001. The null hypothesis is rejected, and we can conclude that, for patients with stage IV lung cancer, there is an association between brain metastases and KPS, with those with brain metastases having a higher risk of KPS less than 70 than those without brain metastases.

CHI-SQUARE TEST VERSUS LOGISTIC REGRESSION

When considering categorical data analysis, it is important to realize that the 2 × 2 tables allow for only two variables to be compared together. The chi-square test can be adapted to consider three variables together in a stratified table context, but researchers are very limited in their abilities to compare relationships of variables in context to other variables. This is where the true strength of logistic regression is shown.

When comparing two variables, logistic regression will give the same results as the 2 × 2 chi-square test. However, logistic regression is not limited to two variables. Logistic regression also does not limit the independent variables. This means the independent variables can be categorical or continuous in nature.

EFFECT SIZE ESTIMATORS

Relative risk and odds ratio are *effect size estimators* used as measures of the relative effect between the groups being compared in a study.

RELATIVE RISK

Relative risk calculations determine the ratio of the probability or likelihood of an event occurring in one group to the probability or likelihood of an event occurring in another group.

Relative risk can be used as an effect size estimator for data analyzed by logistic regression or for data analyzed by a chi-square test. It is much easier to calculate relative risk if the 2 × 2 frequency table has a pre-calculated "Total" row and column.

Example

Going back to the preceding example of the logistic regression, which examines the relationship between breast tumor diameter and risk of involved axillary lymph nodes, we examine the probability of having positive axillary lymph nodes for breast tumor diameters less than or equal to two cm versus greater than two cm.

Tumor Size (cm)	Lymph Node Status (Negative vs. Positive/Yes vs. No)
.4/≤2 cm	Negative/No
.5/≤2 cm	Negative/No
.8/≤2 cm	Negative/No
.8/≤2 cm	Negative/No
.9/≤2 cm	Negative/No
1/≤2 cm	Negative/No
1.1/≤2 cm	Negative/No
1.1/≤2 cm	Negative/No
1.2/≤2 cm	Negative/No
1.3/≤2 cm	Positive/Yes
1.3/≤2 cm	Negative/No

(*continued*)

Tumor Size (cm)	Lymph Node Status (Negative vs. Positive/Yes vs. No)
1.5/≤2 cm	Negative/No
1.7/≤2 cm	Positive/Yes
1.8/≤2 cm	Negative/No
1.8/≤2 cm	Negative/No
1.9/≤2 cm	Positive/Yes
2.1/>2 cm	Negative/No
2.1/>2 cm	Positive/Yes
2.2/>2 cm	Positive/Yes
2.8/>2 cm	Positive/Yes
3.2/>2 cm	Positive/Yes
3.4/>2 cm	Positive/Yes
4.8/>2 cm	Positive/Yes
5.5/>2 cm	Positive/Yes

First, we must construct a 2 × 2 frequency table.

	Dependent Variable Positive	Dependent Variable Negative	Total
Independent variable positive	a	b	$a + b$
Independent variable negative	c	d	$c + d$
Total	$a + c$	$b + d$	$a + b + c + d$

Then we calculate the relative risk using Equation 7.2:

$$\text{Relative Risk} = \frac{\dfrac{a}{a+b}}{\dfrac{c}{c+d}} \tag{7.2}$$

	Lymph Nodes Positive	Lymph Nodes Negative	Total
Tumor size >2 cm	7	1	8
Tumor size ≤2 cm	3	13	16
Total	10	14	24

$$\text{Relative Risk} = \frac{7/8}{3/16} = \frac{.875}{.1875} = 4.67$$

In this dataset, the relative risk or probability of a patient with a tumor greater than two cm having involved lymph nodes is 4.67 times the probability of a patient with a tumor less than or equal to two cm having involved lymph nodes.

ODDS RATIO

Odds ratios are ratios used to measure association between two variables, at least one of which is categorical. Odds ratios can be calculated for data analyzed by logistic regression or a chi-square test. The key to understanding how to calculate an odds ratio is to remember that is a ratio of ODDS. It is important to understand the difference between odds and probability. The difference is best illustrated by the simple concept of rolling a dice. If you have a fair dice, the odds of rolling a 1 are 1:5 (there is one number 1 and there are 5 other numbers [2 – 6]). If you roll the dice 60 times, on average, it is expected that a 1 would be rolled 10 times and another number (not a 1, a 2 – 6) would be rolled 50 times. The probability of rolling a 1 is 1/6.

It will be much easier to remember how you calculate odds ratios if you remember that 2 × 2 frequency tables for odds ratios do not need to have a "Total" row or column.

Example

Again, going back to the previous example of the logistic regression, which examined the relationship between tumor diameter and risk of involved lymph nodes, we examine the odds of having positive lymph nodes for tumor diameter less than or equal to two cm versus greater than two cm.

Tumor Diameter (cm)	Lymph Node Status (Negative vs. Positive/Yes vs. No)
.4/≤2 cm	Negative/No
.5/≤2 cm	Negative/No
.8/≤2 cm	Negative/No
.8/≤2 cm	Negative/No
.9/≤2 cm	Negative/No
1/≤2 cm	Negative/No
1.1/≤2 cm	Negative/No
1.1/≤2 cm	Negative/No
1.2/≤2 cm	Negative/No
1.3/≤2 cm	Positive/Yes
1.3/≤2 cm	Negative/No
1.5/≤2 cm	Negative/No
1.7/≤2 cm	Positive/Yes
1.8/≤2 cm	Negative/No
1.8/≤2 cm	Negative/No
1.9/≤2 cm	Positive/Yes
2.1/>2 cm	Negative/No
2.1/>2 cm	Positive/Yes
2.2/>2 cm	Positive/Yes
2.8/>2 cm	Positive/Yes
3.2/>2 cm	Positive/Yes
3.4/>2 cm	Positive/Yes
4.8/>2 cm	Positive/Yes
5.5/>2 cm	Positive/Yes

First, we must construct a 2 × 2 frequency table.

	Dependent Variable Positive	Dependent Variable Negative
Independent variable positive	a	b
Independent variable negative	c	d

Then we calculate the odds ratio using Equation 7.3.

$$\text{Odds Ratio} = \frac{a/c}{b/d} \qquad (7.3)$$

	Lymph Nodes Positive	Lymph Nodes Negative
Tumor diameter >2 cm	7	1
Tumor diameter ≤2 cm	3	13

$$\text{Odds Ratio} = \frac{7/3}{1/13} = \frac{7*13}{3*1} = \frac{91}{3} = 30.3$$

This means that, based on the dataset used, if you have a tumor greater than two cm, the odds are approximately 30 to 1 that lymph nodes will be involved by cancer.

RELATIVE RISK VERSUS ODDS RATIO

When comparing relative risk versus odds ratio, it is important to understand the most appropriate use of each of these effect size estimators. Cross-sectional studies lend themselves to both relative risk and odds ratios. Cohort studies are best analyzed using relative risk. Case-control studies are most appropriately analyzed by odds ratios. This distinction is rooted in how each of these types of studies is designed. The design of cohort studies, case-control studies, and cross-sectional studies are described in great detail in the Non-Experimental Studies section in Chapter 11. Briefly, the design of cohort studies is based upon categorization by exposure to a risk factor, while the design of case-control studies is based upon categorization by outcome. In a case-control study, the groups are defined on the basis of outcome, and as such, the risk (the probability or chance) of the outcome occurring does not apply; it is somewhat artificial because the probability is determined by how many patients in each group are included as per the study design. The odds ratio is appropriate, however, because it is a comparison of risk versus no risk—not of total events.

Example

Using the preceding example examining the relationship between tumor diameter (≤2 cm vs. >2 cm) and risk of positive lymph node, let us imagine how a cross-sectional, cohort study, and a case-control study would be designed.

A cross-sectional study would simply examine a representative population of women with breast cancer at a given point of time. Diameter of tumor and involvement of axillary lymph nodes would be recorded for all patients. Then, data would be analyzed via cross-sectional regression to determine the relationship between tumor diameter and risk of involved lymph nodes. Relative risk or odds ratio would both be appropriate effect size estimators for this analysis.

A cohort study would compare two groups of women with breast cancer: those with tumors measuring less than or equal to two cm and those with tumors larger than two cm. The risk of involved lymph nodes would be compared between the two groups. In this case, the subjects are grouped according to tumor diameter. Then, the two groups are examined for this incidence of involved lymph nodes. This study design allows the calculation of incidence based upon tumor size (≤2 cm vs. 2 cm) as a risk factor, and thus, the use of relative risk is appropriate.

A case-control study would identify women with breast cancer with positive axillary lymph nodes and women with breast cancer with negative lymph nodes, and compare the two groups to see whether there is a difference in primary tumor diameter (≤2 cm vs. 2 cm) between them. With this case-control design, patients are grouped based on outcome. Thus, the incidence of lymph nodes in each group is artificial; it is not a true incidence because it is determined by the investigators. Without a true incidence, relative risk should not be calculated, and as such, an odds ratio is used to estimate relative risk for a case-control study.

McNEMAR'S TEST

The *McNemar test* is used to analyze data in the 2 × 2 table with paired dichotomous categorical variables.

Example

Let us use the fictional example of a dataset examining the risk of thrombocytopenia before and after treatment with a chemotherapeutic agent. The null hypothesis (H_0) states that the proportion of patients with thrombocytopenia prior to treatment is the same as the proportion of patients with thrombocytopenia after treatment. The raw data for a sample of 30 patients is presented:

Patient Number	Platelet Level Pre-Treatment (×10⁹/L)	Platelet Level After 3 Months of Treatment (×10⁹/L)
1	294	189
2	307	154
3	140	167
4	328	290
5	202	80
6	300	67
7	255	168
8	155	180
9	276	99
10	284	137
11	179	150
12	226	254
13	118	85
14	287	325
15	266	123
16	82	56
17	399	456
18	144	83
19	371	199
20	157	75
21	281	363
22	226	232
23	335	297
24	266	170
25	95	132
26	174	86
27	189	135
28	237	136
29	222	262
30	198	117

To start, the platelet count before and after treatment would need to recorded as a dichotomous nominal variable (thrombocytopenia for platelet count less than $140 \times 10^9/\text{L}$ or not thrombocytopenia for platelet count greater than or equal to $140 \times 10^9/\text{L}$):

Patient Number	Thrombocytopenia Before Treatment	Thrombocytopenia After Treatment
1	No	No
2	No	No
3	No	No
4	No	No
5	No	Yes
6	No	Yes
7	No	No
8	No	No
9	No	Yes
10	No	Yes
11	No	No
12	No	No
13	Yes	Yes
14	No	No
15	No	Yes
16	Yes	Yes
17	No	No
18	No	Yes
19	No	No
20	No	Yes
21	No	No
22	No	No
23	No	No
24	No	No
25	Yes	Yes
26	No	Yes
27	No	Yes
28	No	Yes
29	No	No
30	No	Yes

To analyze the data, we construct a 2 × 2 table:

	Thrombocytopenia After Treatment	No Thrombocytopenia After Treatment	Total
Thrombocytopenia before treatment	3	0	3
No thrombocytopenia before treatment	11	16	27
Total	14	16	30

If there was no association between the chemotherapeutic agent and thrombocytopenia, you would expect each patient with a normal platelet count before treatment to have a normal platelet count after treatment. The number of patients with thrombocytopenia before treatment who recovered after treatment should equal the number of patients with normal platelet counts before receiving treatment who became thrombocytopenic after receiving the agent. For the preceding dataset, there were 11 discordant pairs. There were 11 patients who had normal platelet counts prior to receiving the chemotherapeutic agent who then developed thrombocytopenia after receiving the agent. Conversely, there were no patients who had thrombocytopenia before receiving the chemotherapeutic agent whose platelet counts returned to normal after receiving the agent.

The uncorrected McNemar chi-square statistic equals 11 with a p-value of .009. This corresponds to a continuity-corrected McNemar chi-square statistic of 9.09 and a p-value of .0026. Based on this p-value, we reject the null hypothesis, and conclude that the chemotherapeutic treatment results in a different (in this case, higher) rate of thrombocytopenia.

MANTEL–HAENSZEL METHOD

The *Mantel–Haenszel method* is a technique that generates an estimate of an association between a dichotomous independent variable and a dichotomous dependent variable from multiple datasets collected at separate times or locations or from a slightly different patient population. The data in such a scenario is presented as multiple 2 × 2 tables.

Example

Continuing the previous 2 × 2 table example: we are given KPS as less than 70 or greater than or equal to 70, and information about whether patients have brain metastases or no brain metastases/extracranial disease only.
The following 2 × 2 table was constructed:

	No Brain Metastases/ Extracranial Disease Only	Brain Metastases	Total
KPS <70	104	302	406
KPS ≥70	338	282	620
Total	442	584	1,026

A chi-square test was performed and the p-value was calculated to be less than .0001.

Now, let us imagine that this dataset was collected from a hospital in New York City where patients often come for a second opinion. The mean age of patients in this dataset is 57 years. Let us imagine that there is a second similar dataset collected from patients in a hospital that serves multiple retirement communities in Florida. The average age of patients in this dataset is 72 years old.

A 2 × 2 table is constructed from the dataset collected in Florida:

	No Brain Metastases/ Extracranial Disease Only	Brain Metastases	Total
KPS <70	208	225	433
KPS ≥70	155	161	316
Total	363	368	749

A chi-square test was performed and the chi-square statistic equals .040, which corresponds to a p-value of .8414. One must be cautious in combining these two datasets, because location or age (or some other unidentified factor) may be confounding. This is where the Mantel–Haenszel method is useful.

HOMOGENEITY TEST

A Mantel–Haenszel homogeneity test is used to determine whether the multiple datasets are homogeneous or heterogeneous; that is, if the datasets show similar proportions or independent proportions. The null hypothesis (H_0) states that there is no consistent difference in proportions in the 2 × 2 table constructed from the data obtained in New York City compared to the proportions in the 2 × 2 table constructed from the data obtained in Florida. A Mantel–Haenszel calculator yields a chi-square statistic of 49.3 with 1 degree of freedom and a corresponding p-value of less than .00001. Based on this p-value, we reject the null hypothesis and conclude that there is a significant difference in proportions in the 2 × 2 table constructed from the data obtained in New York City compared to the proportions in the 2 × 2 table constructed from the data obtained in Florida

SUMMARY ODDS RATIO

To be completely correct, the null hypothesis (H_0) of the Mantel–Haenszel test is that the odds ratios from each of the datasets is equal to 1. The Mantel–Haenszel test produces a single, summary measure of association, which provides a weighted average of the odds ratio across the different strata of the confounding factor (location or age in our example).

REFERENCES

1. McMeekin DS, Tritchler DL, Cohn DE, et al. Clinicopathologic significance of mismatch repair defects in endometrial cancer: an NRG oncology/gynecologic oncology. *J Clin Oncol*. 2016;34:3062–3068. doi:10.1200/JCO.2016.67.8722
2. Camilli G, Hopkins K D. Applicability of chi-square to 2 × 2 contingency tables with small expected cell frequencies. *Psychological Bulletin*. 1978;85:163–167. doi:10.1037/0033-2909.85.1.163

Survival Analysis Methods

Survival analysis is the cornerstone of oncologic biostatistics. *Survival analysis* compares time to an event between multiple groups.

TIME-TO-EVENT DATA

Survival analyses use time-to-event data. *Time-to-event data* is different from the other data we have discussed, in that the dependent variable in time-to-event analysis is not just a dichotomous outcome (e.g., survival or recurrence), but also incorporates a temporal element to the outcome (e.g., how long the patient survives or time to recurrence).

KAPLAN–MEIER CURVES

Kaplan–Meier curves are the most basic analysis of time-to-event data.

The goal is that, after reading this chapter, you will be able to do hand calculations for a Kaplan–Meier curve (yes, you will understand the process that well). Honestly, performing such calculations is not necessary as there are Kaplan–Meier calculators available on the Internet and with statistical software. Still, it is critically important for oncologists to understand how these calculations work.

A *Kaplan–Meier curve* measures the fraction of patients living at a specific time after intervention or treatment. The idea is that, if you look at a survival curve for a group of patients who have received a particular treatment, you can predict what percentage of patients would be alive at any given time point.

Hosmer and Lemeshow used a particularly illustrative analogy to explain the Kaplan–Meier estimator:

"This estimator incorporates information from all of the observations available, both uncensored and censored, by considering survival to any point in time as a series of steps defined by the observed survival and censored times. It is analogous to considering a toddler who must take five steps to walk from a chair to a table. This journey of five steps must begin with one successful step. The second step can only be taken if the first was successful. The third step can be taken only if the second (and also the first) was successful. Finally, the fifth step is possible only if the previous four were completed successfully. In an analysis of survival time, we estimated the conditional probabilities of 'successful steps' and them multiply them together to obtain an estimate of the overall survivorship function."(1)

Example

To illustrate Kaplan–Meier survival probabilities, we will use the example of a novel immunotherapy agent being tested in a Phase II trial in patients with metastatic melanoma. Patients with stage IV melanoma without a BRAF mutation who have failed first-line immunotherapy enroll on the trial and are treated with a novel immunotherapy agent. The primary end-point is overall survival. For this small study, the accrual goal is 20 patients. Patients are accrued over a one-year period. An interim analysis of the first 10 patients is performed. The following table details the enrollment date, the date of last follow-up, survival status (dead or alive), and date of death for the first 10 patients enrolled.

The steps to calculate Kaplan–Meier survival probabilities test are as follows:

Kaplan–Meier step 1: Collect date of enrollment, date of last follow-up, survival (or event) status at last follow-up, and date of death (or event):

Patient #	Enrollment Date	Last Follow-up Date	Survival Status	Date of Death
1	01/05/2012	06/17/2013	Alive	
2	01/09/2012	06/03/2013	Alive	
3	02/16/2012	04/03/2013	Deceased	04/03/2013
4	03/02/2012	05/02/2013	Deceased	05/02/2013
5	03/28/2012	09/27/2013	Alive	
6	05/01/2012	02/28/2013	Deceased	02/28/2013
7	05/18/2012	11/12/2013	Alive	
8	05/29/2012	12/02/2013	Alive	
9	06/15/2012	11/10/2013	Deceased	11/10/2013
10	06/25/2012	07/17/2013	Deceased	07/17/2013

To understand this analysis, one must understand the concepts of an event and of censored data. An *event* occurs when a subject experiences the outcome described by the primary endpoint. For overall survival, the event in question is death. For progression free survival, the event in question is either progression of disease or death. A subject is *censored* if he or she has not experienced an event (e.g., if he or she is alive in a study with an overall survival endpoint or if he or she is alive and without disease progression in a study with a progression free survival endpoint), but the last follow-up is shorter than the total study period.

The time interval we will set is one month. Thus, the data (number of patients remaining in the sample either because they are uncensored or alive) will be assessed each month. Thus, the step size in our estimator will be one month.

Kaplan–Meier step 2: Examine data in terms of how many months each patient remains in the data set before being censored or before dying:

Patient #	Number of Months	Censored or Event
1	17	Censored
2	16	Censored
3	11	Event
4	14	Event
5	17	Censored
6	9	Event
7	17	Censored
8	18	Censored
9	16	Event
10	12	Event

Kaplan–Meier step 3: Reorganize the data in order of shortest time to longest time as so:

Patient #	Number of Months	Censored or Event
6	9	Event
3	11	Event
10	12	Event
4	14	Event

(continued)

Patient #	Number of Months	Censored or Event
2	16	Censored
9	16	Event
1	17	Censored
5	17	Censored
7	17	Censored
8	18	Censored

Kaplan–Meier step 4: Examine each time interval, and count the number of patients at risk and the number of deaths:

Time Interval	Number of Patients at Risk Just Before Beginning of the Interval	Number of Deaths During the Interval	Number of Patients CENSORED During the Interval	Number of Patients SURVIVING at the end of the Interval
0–9 months	10	1	0	9
9–11 months	9 alive, none censored	1	0	8
11–12 months	8 alive, none censored	1	0	7
12–14 months	7 alive, none censored	1	0	6
14–16 months	6 alive, none censored	1	1	5
16–17 months	6 − 1 − 1 = 4 5 alive, 1 censored	0	3	4
17–18 months	4 − 0 − 3 = 1 4 alive, 3 censored	0	1	1

Kaplan–Meier step 5: The Kaplan–Meier estimator is then calculated as a probability estimate for each time period (except the first) as a compound conditional probability as follows.

Time Interval	Number of Patients AT RISK Just Before Beginning of Interval	Number of Patients DEATHS During the Interval	Number of Patients CENSORED During the Interval	Number of Patients SURVIVING at the end of the Interval	
0–9 months	10	1	0	9	9/10 = .9
9–11 months	9	1	0	8	(9/10) × (8/9) .9 × .89 = .8
11–12 months	8	1	0	7	(9/10) × (8/9) × (7/8) .9 × .89 × .875 = .7
12–14 months	7	1	0	6	(9/10) × (8/9) × (7/8) × (6/7) .9 × .89 × .875 × .857 = .6
14–16 months	6	1	1	5	(9/10) × (8/9) × (7/8) × (6/7) × (5/6) .9 × .89 × .875 × .857 × .83 = .5
16–17 months	4	0	3	4	(9/10) × (8/9) × (7/8) × (6/7) × (5/6) × (4/4) .9 × .89 × .875 × .857 × .83 × 1 = .5
17–18 months	1	0	1	1	(9/10) × (8/9) × (7/8) × (6/7) × (5/6) × (4/4) × (1/1) .9 × .89 × .875 × .857 × .83 × 1 × 1 = .5

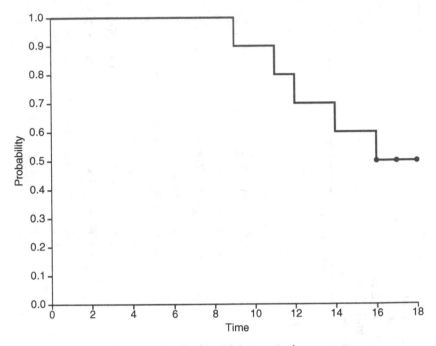

Figure 8.1   Kaplan–Meier survival curve.

The calculated estimate for surviving nine months is 90%. If a patient survives nine months, then the conditional probability (conditional upon having survived the first nine months) of surviving two more months is 89%. Together, these estimates lead us to conclude that the estimated probability of surviving nine months and then surviving another two months is 80% (.90 × .89 = .80). If a patient survives the first 11 months, the conditional probability (conditional upon having survived the first 11 months) of surviving yet another month to 12 months is 87.5%. The estimated probability of surviving 11 months and then surviving another month is, therefore, 70% (.80 × .875 = .70). And, so on.

The data in the preceding table is typically plotted in a survival curve as shown in Figure 8.1.

MEDIAN SURVIVAL

The *median survival* of a Kaplan–Meier survival curve is represented as the time point at which the probability of surviving is 50%. In the preceding dataset, the median survival is approximately 16 months.

Obviously, Kaplan–Meier calculations are complex, and it is not practical to do these by hand, especially for large sample sizes. Thus, these calculations are more practically performed with the available calculator.

LOG-RANK TEST

The *log-rank test* is a test used to compare time-to-event data between two groups.

Carrying over the example of the novel immunotherapy agent in BRAF mutation negative metastatic melanoma, the log-rank test would be used in analysis of a randomized Phase II or Phase III trial. In such a trial, patients with stage IV melanoma without a BRAF mutation who have failed first-line immunotherapy would be randomized to treatment either with placebo or with a novel immunotherapy agent. Patients would be followed for a minimum of two years, and survival would be the primary endpoint. Time-to-event (death) data would be recorded.

The log-rank test is used to test the null hypothesis (H_0) that there is no difference in the time to a particular event between two groups. For our example, the null hypothesis (H_0) would be that there is no difference in the survival curves for patients treated with placebo and those treated with the novel immunotherapy agent. This log-rank analysis takes into account not only deaths, but also censored events.

The log-rank test is most commonly used to compare Kaplan–Meier curves between two groups. The log-rank test should be used to compare groups in which data observations have been censored.

Example

To demonstrate the log-rank test, we will adapt the example used to demonstrate the Kaplan–Meier curve earlier. Imagine that the 10 patients with stage IV melanoma without a BRAF mutation who have failed first-line immunotherapy and have received the novel immunotherapy agent comprise the experimental arm of a Phase III randomized trial comparing the novel immunotherapy agent (Arm A) to placebo (Arm B). Imagine that we are performing an interim analysis of the first 10 patients treated in each group. The null hypothesis (H_0) states that there is no difference in survival between those receiving the novel immunotherapy agent and those receiving placebo. The alpha level is set at .05.

The data are presented as follows:

Patient Number	Number of Months	Censored or Event	Group
1	17	Censored	A – Novel agent
2	16	Censored	A – Novel agent

(continued)

Patient Number	Number of Months	Censored or Event	Group
3	11	Event	A – Novel agent
4	14	Event	A – Novel agent
5	17	Censored	A – Novel agent
6	9	Event	A – Novel agent
7	17	Censored	A – Novel agent
8	18	Censored	A – Novel agent
9	16	Event	A – Novel agent
10	12	Event	A – Novel agent

Patient Number	Number of Months	Censored or Event	Group
11	9	Event	B – Placebo
12	5	Event	B – Placebo
13	14	Event	B – Placebo
14	9	Event	B – Placebo
15	11	Event	B – Placebo
16	3	Censored	B – Placebo
17	10	Censored	B – Placebo
18	8	Event	B – Placebo
19	6	Censored	B – Placebo
20	10	Event	B – Placebo

The log-rank test calculator is used to calculate a p-value of .0038. As the p-value is less than the predetermined alpha level, the null hypothesis is rejected.

The log-rank test is visualized as a comparison of Kaplan–Meier curves of the two groups in Figure 8.2.

WILCOXON RANK-SUM TEST

If censored observations are not present in the data, then the Wilcoxon rank-sum test is the appropriate test.

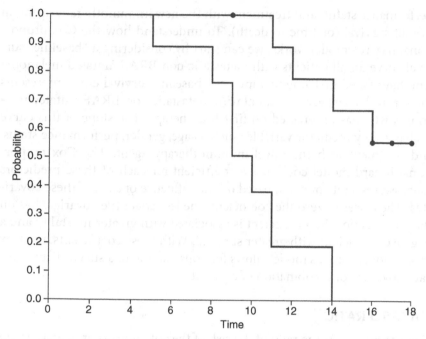

Figure 8.2 Survival curves comparing group A and group B using the log-rank test.

COX PROPORTIONAL HAZARDS MODEL

The *Cox proportional hazards model* is a survival model that analyzes time-to-event data, and also accounts for the effect of covariates. The Kaplan–Meier method and log-rank test described are used to compare survival curves among groups, but the Cox proportional hazards model takes the analysis further in allowing to analyze the effects of several factors on survival in those groups.

Covariates analyzed via a Cox proportional hazards model can be categorical or continuous. The Cox proportional hazards model is a regression that allows us to assess the effect of covariate predictors on the shape of the survival curve.

Example

Expanding further upon the example of the use of a novel immunotherapy agent in patients with non-BRAF mutated metastatic melanoma who have failed first-line therapy, let us consider the impact of patient age, gender, performance status, and treatment with the new immunotherapy agent on overall survival (or time to death). To understand how the Cox proportional hazards model works, we can start by considering a "baseline" survival curve for all patients with metastatic non-BRAF mutated melanoma who have failed first-line therapy. This baseline survival curve represents the survival of an average patient with metastatic non-BRAF mutated melanoma who has progressed on first-line therapy. The slope of this curve is changed by predictor variables such as age, gender, performance status, and treatment with the novel immunotherapy agent. The Cox proportional hazard model computes a coefficient for each of these predictors that assesses a rate of death based on the influence of each of these covariates. The closer to zero the coefficient, the less effect the covariate has on the curve. A positive coefficient is associated with greater mortality and a negative coefficient with greater survival. With these coefficients, the Cox proportional hazards model allows for construction of a survival curve for each covariate or combination of covariates.

HAZARD RATIO

The *hazard ratio* is the ratio of the risk of the outcome event over a certain period of time for different categories of covariates as determined from the Cox proportional hazards model. The hazard ratio should be interpreted as the chance of an event occurring in the treatment arm divided by the chance of the event occurring in the control arm, or vice versa, over the full-time course of the study. For example, if at the end of study period, 25% of the patients who received placebo are alive and 50% of patients who received the novel immunotherapy agent are alive, the hazard ratio of death for those receiving placebo would be two.

From the perspective of hypothesis testing, for each covariate, the null hypothesis (H_0) is that the covariate has no effect on survival or that the hazard ratio for the covariate = 1. For each covariate that impacts the Cox proportional hazards curve with an associated *p*-value less than alpha, the null hypothesis (H_0) will be rejected.

Calculations for the Cox proportional hazards model are quite complex and beyond the scope of this text. These calculations are best carried out using a Cox proportional hazards model calculator.

REFERENCE

1. Hosmer D, Lemeshow S. *Applied Survival Analysis: Regression Modeling of Time-to-event Data* (1st ed.), Wiley; 1999.

Guide to Choosing the Appropriate Statistical Test

The following table provides a guide to the most appropriate statistical test to use for a given analysis based on the type and number of independent and dependent variables:

				Type of dependent variable		
				Quantitative	Qualitative	Time-to-event
Type of independent variable	Qualitative	Comparing two groups	Unpaired	Independent t-test	Chi-square test or Fisher's exact test	Log-rank test or Cox-proportional hazards regression
			Paired	Paired t-test		
		Comparing >3 groups	Unpaired	ANOVA		
			Paired	ANOVA		
	Quantitative	1 independent variable		Simple linear regression or correlation	Logistic regression	Cox proportional hazards regression
		>2 independent variables		Multiple linear regression		

Most of the examples of studies that we have used thus far and most of the examples of clinical trials that will be used in Section III are examples of superiority analyses. Many clinical trials in oncology are designed as non-inferiority analyses. Noninferiority trials are appropriate if an investigator would like to introduce a novel intervention that has some established advantage over the standard of care (less expensive, more convenient, better tolerated). In order for this novel intervention to be accepted as the new standard of care, the investigator must prove that the novel intervention is not unacceptably less effective than the standard of care.

A properly designed noninferiority analysis incorporates clinical judgment to determine a noninferiority margin. The null hypothesis (H_0) for a noninferiority trial states that the novel intervention is inferior in efficacy to the standard of care by a difference more than the pre-determined non-inferiority margin. The alternative hypothesis states that the novel intervention is not inferior in efficacy to the standard of care by more than the pre-determined noninferiority margin.

Example

The TARGIT-A trial investigating intraoperative radiotherapy for early-stage breast cancer is an example of a noninferiority trial in oncology (1). In total, 1,721 patients with early-stage breast cancer in this trial were randomized to fractionated whole breast external beam radiotherapy (EBRT) following surgery versus single-dose targeted intraoperative radiotherapy (TARGIT). The primary outcome was absolute difference in local recurrence in the conserved breast, with a prescribed noninferiority margin of 2.5% at five years. The alpha value was set at .01 for local recurrence.

The null hypothesis (H_0) in this study states that TARGIT is inferior to EBRT in terms of local recurrence by more than the margin of 2.5%. The alternative hypothesis is that TARGIT is noninferior to EBRT in terms of local recurrence. TARGIT is given in a single fraction and is, therefore, significantly more convenient than the standard protracted course of EBRT.

Totally, 23 or 3.3% of the patients in the TARGIT arm and 11 or 1.3% of the patients in the EBRT experienced local recurrence. The absolute difference in recurrence rate between the two groups was 2%. The log-rank test was used to compare time to local recurrence between the two groups. The p-value for this log-rank test analysis was .042. The p-value for local recurrence comparison was greater than the pre-established alpha value of .01. Thus, the null hypothesis (H_0) was not rejected. However, the authors of publication point out that the difference in local control (2%) was less than the pre-determined noninferiority margin of 2.5%. The statistical design and conclusions of the TARGIT publication have been scrutinized and commented upon in other publications (2). The appropriate use of the noninferiority criterion would be to declare noninferiority only if the upper confidence interval (CI) is less than the pre-defined noninferiority margin. Unfortunately, the CI for this log-rank test was not provided, so ultimately, the appropriate statistical conclusion cannot be confirmed.

Statistical literature has commented that noninferiority trials reward the careless investigator (3). Noninferiority trials are also subject to a lack of assay sensitivity.

REFERENCES

1. Vaidya JS, Wenz F, Bulsara M, et al. Risk-adapted targeted intraoperative radiotherapy versus whole-breast radiotherapy for breast cancer: 5-year results for local control and overall survival from the TARGIT-A randomized trial. *Lancet*. 2014;383:603–613. doi:10.1016/S0140-6736(13)61950-9
2. Cuzik J. Radiotherapy for breast cancer, the TARGIT-A trial. *Lancet*. 2014;383:1716. doi:10.1016/S0140-6736(14)60825-4
3. Schumi J, Wittes JT. Through the looking glass: understanding noninferiority. *Trials*. 2011;12:106–117. doi:10.1186/1745-6215-12-106

HYPOTHESIS TESTING

1. An oncologist has been investigating side effects of a new chemotherapeutic agent. Preclinical data suggests that the agent is associated with thrombocytopenia. The physician collects platelet levels from 30 patients prior to receiving this medication and platelet levels from the same 30 patients after they have been receiving the chemotherapeutic agent for three months.

   The data is presented as follows:

Patient Number	Platelet Level Pre-Treatment ($\times 10^9$/L)	Platelet Level After Three Months of Treatment ($\times 10^9$/L)
1	294	189
2	307	154
3	140	167
4	328	290
5	202	80
6	300	67
7	255	168
8	155	180
9	276	99
10	284	137
11	179	150
12	226	254
13	118	85
14	287	325
15	266	123

(continued)

Patient Number	Platelet Level Pre-Treatment (×10⁹/L)	Platelet Level After Three Months of Treatment (×10⁹/L)
16	82	56
17	399	456
18	144	83
19	371	199
20	157	75
21	281	363
22	226	232
23	335	297
24	266	170
25	95	132
26	174	86
27	189	135
28	237	136
29	222	262
30	198	117

a. What is the null hypothesis?

b. What is the appropriate statistical test?

c. If the value of α is set at .05 and β is 30%, what is the probability of Type I error?

d. If the value of α is set at .05 and β is 30%, what is the probability of Type II error?

e. What is the probability of rejecting a null hypothesis that is true?

f. What is the probability of not rejecting a null hypothesis that is false?

g. What is the statistical power?

h. What is the mean of each sample?

i. What is the standard deviation of each sample?

j. Calculate the p-value for the comparison and determine whether to reject H_0.

k. State the conclusion in words.

2. Researchers are conducting a Phase II randomized trial of a PDL-1 inhibitor in patients with metastatic non-small cell lung cancer (NSCLC) who have progressed on cytotoxic chemotherapy and whose tumors express PDL-1. A total of 83 patients are enrolled in the trial; 43 are randomized to receive the novel agent and 40 are randomized to receive placebo. In Phase I clinical trials, the most common side effect seen with the PDL-1 inhibitor was pneumonitis. With a median follow-up of 11 months, five patients in the PDL-1 inhibitor group and zero patients in the placebo group have developed clinical pneumonitis. The researches aim to determine whether the development of pneumonitis is the result of chance or whether it is related to the PDL-1 inhibitor.

   a. What is the most appropriate test to compare the proportion of patients who developed pneumonitis in the PDL-1 group versus in the placebo group?

   b. What is the null hypothesis for this test?

   c. A test for binomial proportions reveals that the p-value for the comparison between the two groups is .03. If the alpha level is set at .05, what is the hypothesis testing conclusion?

3. A retrospective research study is conducted to compare the mean tumor diameter for patients with stage I-II lung cancer treated with lobectomy versus stereotactic body radiotherapy (SBRT). There are 20 patients in each group. The tumor diameter for each group is as follows:

Patient Number	SBRT Cohort Mean Tumor Diameter (cm)	Lobectomy Cohort Mean Tumor Diameter (cm)
1	2.3	1.9
2	1.7	2.5
3	1.4	2.4
4	2.8	2.9
5	2.2	1.8
6	3.0	2.6
7	3.5	2.2
8	3.1	1.8
9	2.7	2.9
10	2.8	2.4

(continued)

Patient Number	SBRT Cohort Mean Tumor Diameter (cm)	Lobectomy Cohort Mean Tumor Diameter (cm)
11	1.8	1.5
12	2.3	2.5
13	1.8	2.8
14	2.7	3.3
15	2.6	2.0
16	2.8	2.6
17	3.9	4.1
18	1.4	2.8
19	3.1	1.9
20	2.1	3.7

a. What is the difference between the mean of the two groups?

b. What is the standard error of the difference between the two groups?

c. What is the 95% confidence interval of the difference?

d. What p-value level does the 95% confidence interval correspond to?

e. Would the difference between the tumor diameter of these two groups be statistically significant at this level?

f. What is the 99% confidence interval of the difference?

g. What p-value level does the 99% confidence interval correspond to?

h. Would the difference between the tumor diameter of these two groups be statistically significant at this level?

SENSITIVITY AND SPECIFICITY CONCEPTS

1. Yearly low-dose screening chest CT scan for patients with significant smoking history is recommended by the National Comprehensive Cancer Network. This recommendation is based upon the results of a randomized trial by the National Lung Screening Trial Research Team with initial notes published in the *New England Journal of Medicine* in 2013 (1).

   The study included a total of 53,439 eligible participants. 26,715 were randomized to low-dose CT and 26,309 of those underwent screening. Totally, 26,724 were randomized to chest radiography and 26,035 of those underwent screening.

   A total of 7,191 participants in the low-dose CT group and 2,387 in the radiography group had a positive screening result. Lung cancer was diagnosed in 292 participants in the low-dose CT group versus 190 in the radiography group. Totally, 270 of the 292 patients in the low-dose CT group had positive CT scan and the other 18 did not (4 did not show for testing). Totally, 136 of the 190 patients in the radiography group had a positive chest x-ray and 49 did not (5 did not show for testing).

   a. Construct a 2 × 2 table for sensitivity and specificity calculations for low-dose chest CT scan using the patients who underwent testing. Do the same for chest radiography.

   b. When you are calculating the sensitivity and specificity of a test, what value is in the denominator?

   c. What are the sensitivity and specificity of low-dose CT scan and radiology for detection of lung cancer in patients with smoking history?

   d. Which is more sensitive, low-dose CT scan or chest x-ray?

   e. Which is more specific, low-dose CT scan or chest x-ray?

   f. When you are calculating the positive and negative predictive value of a test, what value is in the denominator?

   g. What is the positive predictive value of low-dose CT scan?

   h. What is the negative predictive value of low-dose CT scan?

   i. What is the positive likelihood ratio for low-dose CT scan?

   j. What is the negative likelihood ratio for low-dose CT scan?

REFERENCE

1. NLSTRT. Results of initial low-dose computed tomographic screening for lung cancer. *N Engl J Med*. 2013;368:1980–1989. doi:10.1056/ NEJMoa1209120

CORRELATION AND REGRESSION CONCEPTS

1. What is the main difference between a correlation and a regression?

2. What is the main difference between a linear and logistic regression?

3. A urologist is reviewing the data from the cases of prostate cancer on which he has operated over the past five years. He is interested in studying whether there is a relationship between prostate size (g) and risk of postoperative complications following radical prostatectomy. He considers prostate size (g) the independent variable and the presence of postoperative complications following radical prostatectomy the dependent variable.

   The following is the data from a representative sample of 20 patients:

Prostate Size (g)	Presence of Postoperative Complications (Yes vs. No)
44	No
65	No
48	No
38	No
39	No
50	No
51	No
42	No
52	No
60	Yes
42	No
28	No
77	Yes
48	No
66	No
69	Yes

(continued)

Prostate Size (g)	Presence of Postoperative Complications (Yes vs.No)
90	Yes
33	No
46	Yes
83	Yes

a. What is the most appropriate test to analyze this data?
   a. Pearson correlation
   b. Spearman correlation
   c. Linear regression
   d. Logistic regression
b. What is the null hypothesis for this analysis?
c. Use the appropriate calculator to determine the p-value for this analysis and to determine whether to reject or not reject the null hypothesis if the value of α is set at .05.

4. The same surgeon decides to undertake a similar analysis to examine the relationship between prostate size (g) and number of postoperative complications ($n = 1, 2, 3, 4, \ldots n$) after radical prostatectomy.
   The following is the data from a representative sample of 20 patients:

Prostate Size (g)	Number of Postoperative Complications
44	0
65	0
48	0
38	0
39	0
50	0
51	0
42	0
52	0
60	2
42	0

(continued)

Prostate Size (g)	Number of Postoperative Complications
28	0
77	3
48	0
66	0
69	1
90	1
33	0
46	5
83	2

a. If the surgeon determines that both the prostate size and number of postoperative complications following radical prostatectomy are independent variables, what is the most appropriate test to analyze this data (assume a linear relationship)?

   a. Pearson correlation

   b. Spearman correlation

   c. Linear regression

   d. Logistic regression

b. What is the calculated correlation coefficient?

c. Is this a positive or negative correlation?

d. What is the coefficient of determination?

e. If the surgeon determines prostate size is the independent variable and number of postoperative complications following radical prostatectomy is the dependent variable, what is the most appropriate test to analyze this data.

   a. Pearson correlation

   b. Spearman correlation

   c. Linear regression

   d. Logistic regression

f. What is regression line equation for this analysis?

CATEGORICAL DATA ANALYSIS

1. What is the difference between Fisher's exact test and chi-square test?

2. According to this text, when might it be appropriate to use Fisher's exact test instead of the chi-square test?

3. A clinical researcher trained in hematology/oncology is interested to determine whether there is an association between HPV+ oropharyngeal cancer and the presence of greater than or equal to N3 disease in patients with oropharyngeal cancer. She pools data from multiple institutions comprising a total of 2,837 patients with oropharyngeal cancer. Of these patients, 1,938 patients have documented HPV+ pathology and 899 patients have HPV– pathology. Of the 1,938 patients with HPV+ pathology, 549 have N3 disease. Of the 899 patients with HPV– pathology, 99 patients have N3 disease.

   a. Develop a 2×2 contingency table for this data.

   b. What is the null hypothesis for this researcher's analysis?

   c. Using a hand calculation or a chi-square test calculator, determine the chi-square statistic and p-value for this analysis.

   d. What is the appropriate conclusion of hypothesis testing for this analysis if the value of α is set at .01?

   e. In this study, the researcher identified patients with oropharyngeal cancer and classified those patients according to HPV status (risk factor). The researcher then retrospectively reviewed their charts to determine the clinical N stage. This is an example of what type of study?

   f. What is the appropriate effects size estimator?

   g. Calculate the relative risk of cN3 disease for those with HPV+ versus HPV– disease.

4. The same investigator decides to carry out the same study with a slightly different method. The researcher identifies all of the cases of N3 oropharyngeal cancer treated at the cooperative institutions. A total of 648 patients with clinical N3 oropharyngeal cancer are identified. She identifies a control group of 2,189 patients with clinical N0 to N2 oropharyngeal cancer. She then determines the HPV status of the pathology specimens of each of these patients. A 2 × 2 table is constructed as follows:

	<N3 Disease	N3 Disease
HPV+	1389	549
HPV−	800	99

a. What type of retrospective study has this researcher carried out?

b. What is the appropriate effects size estimator?

c. Calculate the odds ratio of cN3 disease for those with HPV+ versus HPV− disease.

TIME-TO-EVENT ANALYSIS

1. A Phase II clinical trial is being conducted to test a new therapy for renal cell carcinoma. The study has enrolled 30 patients with metastatic renal cell carcinoma who have failed first-line therapy. They are followed a total of five years with a primary outcome of disease-free survival.

   a. What time-to-event data should be recorded in order to calculate disease-free survival (consider the date of enrollment as the start time)?

   b. Reformat the following table/spreadsheet with the necessary information to construct a Kaplan–Meier curve for disease free-survival (DFS).

Patient Number	Enrollment Date	Disease Progression (Y/N)	Date of Disease Progression	Alive (Y/N)	Date of Death	Date of Last Follow-up	Time (Months) to Last Follow-up
1	05/16/2014	Y	11/30/2014	N	04/04/2016	04/04/2016	23
2	07/07/2014	Y	03/27/2015	N	04/24/2016	04/24/2016	22
3	09/19/2014	Y	07/19/2015	N	12/29/2015	12/29/2015	15
4	10/13/2014	Y	04/08/2015	N	01/15/2015	01/15/2015	3
5	11/8/2014	Y	04/29/2015	Y		09/30/2016	23
6	12/03/2014	Y	06/06/2015	Y		09/05/2016	21
7	12/12/2014	Y	09/15/2015	N	06/05/2016	06/05/2016	18
8	01/15/2015	Y	06/17/2016	Y		09/17/2016	20
9	02/16/2015	Y	12/09/2015	N	04/18/2016	04/18/2016	14
10	03/6/2015	Y	01/18/2016	Y		07/18/2016	16
11	04/07/2015	Y	06/23/2016	Y		09/23/2016	18
12	04/23/2015	Y	09/29/2016	N	09/29/2016	09/29/2016	17
13	5/3/2015	Y	12/28/2015	Y		9/28/2016	17
14	06/18/2015	N		Y		09/14/2016	15
15	06/23/2015	Y	03/31/2016	Y		09/30/2016	15
16	07/26/2015	N		N	01/18/2016	01/18/2016	6
17	08/19/2015	Y	09/5/2016	Y		09/5/2016	13

(continued)

Patient Number	Enrollment Date	Disease Progression (Y/N)	Date of Disease Progression	Alive (Y/N)	Date of Death	Date of Last Follow-up	Time (Months) to Last Follow-up
18	09/23/2015	Y	06/07/2016	Y		09/07/2016	11
19	10/11/2015	Y	05/05/2016	N	08/05/2016	08/05/2016	10
20	10/15/2015	N		N	09/04/2016	09/04/2016	11
21	12/01/2015	Y	06/07/2016	Y		09/07/2016	9
22	01/23/2016	Y	05/31/2016	Y		08/31/2016	7
23	02/22/2016	N		Y		09/09/2016	7
24	3/3/2016	Y	8/30/2016	Y		8/30/2016	6
25	03/27/2016	N		Y		09/01/2016	5
26	04/14/2016	N		Y		09/19/2016	5
27	04/25/2016	Y	07/09/2016	N	09/19/2016	09/19/2016	5
28	07/17/2016	N		Y		09/09/2016	2
29	08/09/2016	N		Y		09/11/2016	1
30	08/18/2016	N		Y		09/20/2016	1

c. What is the median DFS?

d. Develop the Kaplan–Meier curve for DFS.

e. How would the spreadsheet for the data differ if you were calculating overall survival? Create the appropriate data spreadsheet for overall survival.

f. What is the median survival?

g. Develop the Kaplan–Meier curve for overall survival.

h. What test should the researcher use if she wishes to investigate the effects of the investigational therapy on DFS in patients younger than 65 years compared to those 65 years and older?

i. What test should the researcher use if she wishes to investigate the effect of age (as a continuous variable), gender, and race on the DFS of patients in this study?

2. **For analysis of overall survival in a randomized Phase III clinical trial comparing an investigational drug to the standard of care, a researcher uses a Cox proportional hazards model to compare survival between the two arms studied while accounting for covariates. A hazard ratio (HR) is calculated as .67 for the experimental arm.**

a. State what the HR of .67 for the experimental group means.

b. What is the HR for the standard of care group?

c. State what the HR of 1.49 for the standard of care group means.

3. **Identify the appropriate statistical test to use for each of the following clinical question scenarios:**

a. How does the hemoglobin of patients change with their age?

b. Which factors influence whether or not a woman with Stage III breast cancer is cured (alive or not alive)?

i. Multiple independent variables (continuous and categorical) and categorical dependent variable

ii. Multiple independent variables (categorical) and binary dependent variable

c. What is the difference in overall survival between men and women?

d. Which factors influence how long a woman with metastatic breast cancer lives?

Section II Problem Set Solutions

HYPOTHESIS TESTING

1.

  a. There is no difference between the mean platelet level before treatment and the mean platelet level after treatment:

$$H_0 : \mu_d = 0$$

  b. Paired t-test

  c. 5%

  d. 30%

  e. 5%

  f. 30%

  g. 70%

  h. Pre-treatment: 233

    Post-treatment: 176

  i. Pre-treatment: 80

    Post-treatment: 97

  j. $p = .0005$. Reject the null hypothesis (H_0).

  k. We conclude that, on average, the platelet level after three months of treatment is lower than the pre-treatment platelet level.

2.

  a. Test of binomial proportions.

  b. The null hypothesis is that there is no difference in the proportion of patients who develop pneumonitis in the PDL-1 group versus the placebo group.

  c. There is a statistically significant difference in the proportion of patients who develop pneumonitis in the PDL-1 group versus the placebo group. Therefore, we reject the null hypothesis.

3.

   a. −0.03

   b. Standard error of the difference = .21

   c. Calculated 95% CI = −.03 +/− 1.96(.21) = (−.44, .38). (Note: 95% CI calculator may yield a result of (−.46, .40)).

   d. 95% CI corresponds to a p-value of .05.

   e. No, the difference between the tumor diameter of these two groups would not be statistically significant at this level because the confidence interval crosses 0.

   f. Calculated 95% CI = −.03 +/− 2.58(.21) = (−.57, .51). (Note: 99%CI calculator may yield a result of (−.60, .54)).

   g. 99% CI corresponds to a p-value of .01.

   h. No, the difference between the tumor diameter of these two groups would not be statistically significant at this level because the confidence interval crosses 0.

SENSITIVITY AND SPECIFICITY CONCEPTS

1.

a.

	Presence of Lung Cancer		
	Positive	**Negative**	**Total**
CT scan	a	b	
Positive	270	6,921	7,191
	c	d	
Negative	18 (+ 4 patients who missed testing)	19,096	19,118
Total	288 (+ 4 patients who missed testing)	26,017	26,309

	Presence of Lung Cancer		
	Positive	**Negative**	**Total**
Radiography	a	b	
Positive	136	2,2511	2,387
	c	d	
Negative	49 (+ 5 patients who missed testing)	23,594	23,648
Total	185 (+ 5 patients who missed testing)	25,845	26,035

b. For calculation of sensitivity and specificity, the denominator is the presence or absence of the disease.

c. SENSITIVITY of low-dose CT scan = $a/(a + c) = 270/288 = 93.8\%$
SPECIFICITY of low-dose CT scan = $d/(b + d) = 19096/26017 = 73.4\%$

d. The low-dose chest CT scan is more sensitive (93.8% vs. 73.4%).

e. The chest x-ray is more specific (91.3% vs. 73.5%).

f. For calculation of positive and negative predictive value the denominator is the result of the test.

g. PPV of low-dose CT scan = Positive predictive value (PPV) = $a/(a + b) = 270/7191 = 3.75\%$

h. NPV of low-dose CT scan = Negative predictive value (NPV) = $d/(c + d) = 19096/19118 = 99.9\%$

i. Positive likelihood ratio for low-dose CT scan = (sensitivity)/(1 − specificity) = $.938/(1 − .734) = 3.53$

j. Negative likelihood ratio for low-dose CT scan = (1 − sensitivity)/(specificity) = $(1 − .938)/.734 = .08$

CORRELATION AND REGRESSION CONCEPTS

1. The main difference between a correlation and a regression is that a correlation involves multiple independent variables, whereas a regression involves at least one dependent variable.

2. The main difference between a linear and logistic regression is the dependent variable. For a linear regression, the dependent variable is a continuous variable, and for a logistic regression, the dependent variable is a categorical variable

3.

   a. **d) Logistic regression** because there is a dependent variable and the dependent variable is binary (presence or absence of postoperative complications).

   b. Null hypothesis (H_0): The probability of surgical complications from radical prostatectomy is not associated with prostate size.

   c. Per logistic regression calculator: Overall model fit: $p = .0208$. Based on this, we reject the null hypothesis and conclude that the probability of surgical complications from radical prostatectomy is associated with prostate size.

4.

   a. **a) Pearson correlation** because there are two independent variables and the relationship is assumed to be linear.

   b. $r = .366$

   c. Positive correlation, because r has a positive value, indicating that as the independent variable increases, so does the dependent variable.

   d. $r^2 = .134$

   e. **c) Linear regression** because the dependent variable is continuous.

   f. Per the linear regression calculator, the regression line equation:

   $$y = .029x + .87.$$

CATEGORICAL DATA ANALYSIS

1. **Fisher's exact test gives an exact p-value and the chi-square test gives an estimate of the p-value.**

2. **It is appropriate to use Fisher's exact test when the total sample size is less than 1,000.**

3.
   a.

	<N3 Disease	N3 Disease	Total
HPV+	1,389	549	1,938
HPV−	800	99	899
Total	2,189	648	2,837

   b. Null hypothesis (H_0): There is no association between HPV positivity and the risk of greater than or equal to clinical N3 disease.
   c. Chi-square = 104.5; df = 1; p-value less than .0001; Corrected chi-square = 103.5; df = 1; p-value less than .0001
   d. Because p-value is less than alpha, we reject the null hypothesis and conclude that there exists an association between HPV positivity and the risk of greater than or equal to clinical N3 disease.
   e. This is an example of a retrospective cohort study.
   f. Relative risk is the appropriate effect size estimator.
   g. Relative risk = $(a/(a + b))/(c/(c + d))$

For this example, you are looking for the risk of N3 disease, so you would reverse the <N3 and N3 columns for this calculation:

	N3 Disease	<N3 Disease	Total
HPV+	549	1,389	1,938
HPV-	99	800	899
Total	648	2,189	2,837

RR = (549/1938)/(99/899) = (.2833)/(.1101) = 2.57

4.
   a. This is a case-control study.
   b. Odds ratio is the appropriate effect size estimator.
   c. Odds ratio = $(a/c)/(b/d) = ad/cb$.

For this example, you are looking for the risk of greater than or equal to N3 disease, so you would reverse the <N3 and ≥N3 columns for this calculation:

	N3 disease	<N3 disease
HPV+	549	1,389
HPV−	99	800

$OR = (549/99)/(1389/800) = (549 \times 800)/(99 \times 1389) = 4{,}392{,}000/137{,}511$
$= 3.19$

TIME-TO-EVENT ANALYSIS

1.
   a. The time from enrollment to evidence of disease progression, new primary cancer, or death (whichever comes first) should be recorded.
   b. The following table/spreadsheet contains the necessary information to construct a Kaplan–Meier curve for DFS:

Patient Number	Enrollment Date	Disease Progression (Y/N)	Date of Disease Progression	Time (Months) to Progression	Alive (Y/N)	Date of Death	Time (Months) to Death	Date of Last Follow-up	Time (Months) to Last Follow-up	Event (1) or Censor (0)	Time-to-Event or Censor
1	05/16/2014	Y	11/30/2014	6	N	04/04/2016	23	04/04/2016	23	1	6
2	07/07/2014	Y	03/27/2015	9	N	04/24/2016	22	04/24/2016	22	1	9
3	09/19/2014	Y	07/19/2015	10	N	12/29/2015	15	12/29/2015	15	1	10
4	10/13/2014	Y	04/08/2015	6	N	01/15/2015	3	01/15/2015	3	1	6
5	11/08/2014	Y	04/29/2015	6	Y			09/30/2016	23	1	6
6	12/03/2014	Y	06/06/2015	6	Y			09/05/2016	21	1	6
7	12/12/2014	Y	09/15/2015	9	N	06/05/2016	18	06/05/2016	18	1	9
8	01/15/2015	Y	06/17/2016	17	Y			09/17/2016	20	1	17
9	02/16/2015	Y	12/09/2015	10	N	04/18/2016	14	04/18/2016	14	1	10
10	03/06/2015	Y	01/18/2016	10	Y			07/18/2016	16	1	10
11	04/07/2015	Y	06/23/2016	15	Y			09/23/2016	18	1	15
12	04/23/2015	Y	09/29/2016	17	N	09/29/2016	17	09/29/2016	17	1	17
13	05/03/2015	Y	12/28/2015	8	Y			09/28/2016	17	1	8
14	06/18/2015	N			Y			09/14/2016	15	0	15
15	06/23/2015	Y	03/31/2016	9	Y			09/30/2016	15	1	9
16	07/26/2015	N			N	01/18/2016	6	01/18/2016	6	1	6
17	08/19/2015	Y	09/05/2016	13	Y			09/05/2016	13	1	13

(continued)

Patient Number	Enrollment Date	Disease Progression (Y/N)	Date of Disease Progression	Time (Months) to Progression	Alive (Y/N)	Date of Death	Time (Months) to Death	Date of Last Follow-up	Time (Months) to Last Follow-up	Event (1) or Censor (0)	Time-to-Event or Censor
18	09/23/2015	Y	06/07/2016	8	Y			09/07/2016	11	1	8
19	10/11/2015	Y	05/05/2016	7	N	08/05/2016		08/05/2016	10	1	7
20	10/15/2015	N			N	09/04/2016	11	09/04/2016	11	1	11
21	12/01/2015	Y	06/07/2016	6	Y			09/07/2016	9	1	6
22	01/23/2016	Y	05/31/2016	4	Y			08/31/2016	7	1	4
23	02/22/2016	N			Y			09/09/2016	7	0	7
24	03/03/2016	Y	08/30/2016	6	Y			08/30/2016	6	1	6
25	03/27/2016	N			Y			09/01/2016	5	0	5
26	04/14/2016	N			Y			09/19/2016	5	0	5
27	04/25/2016	Y	7/9/2016	2	N	09/19/2016	5	09/19/2016	5	1	2
28	07/17/2016	N			Y			09/09/2016	2	0	2
29	08/09/2016	N			Y			09/11/2016	1	0	1
30	08/18/2016	N			Y			09/20/2016	1	0	1

c. Median DFS ~ 8 months

d. Kaplan–Meier curve for DFS:

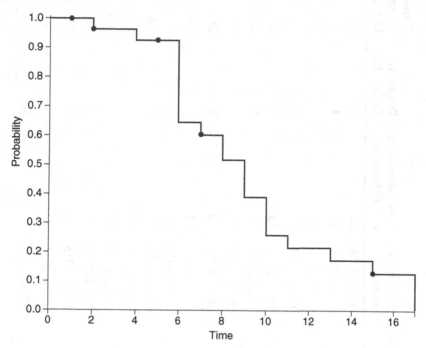

e. How would the spreadsheet for the data differ if you were calculating overall survival? Create the appropriate data spreadsheet for overall survival.

Patient Number	Enrollment Date	Alive (Y/N)	Date of Death	Time (Months) to Death	Date of Last Follow-up	Time (Months) to Last Follow-up	Event (1) or Censor (0)	Time-to-Event or Censor
1	05/16/2014	N	04/04/2016	23	04/04/2016	23	1	23
2	07/07/2014	N	04/24/2016	22	04/24/2016	22	1	22
3	09/19/2014	N	12/29/2015	15	12/29/2015	15	1	15
4	10/13/2014	N	01/15/2015	3	01/15/2015	3	1	3
5	11/08/2014	Y			09/30/2016	23	0	23
6	12/03/2014	Y			09/05/2016	21	0	21
7	12/12/2014	N	06/05/2016	18	06/05/2016	18	1	18
8	01/15/2015	Y			09/17/2016	20	0	20
9	02/16/2015	N	04/18/2016	14	04/18/2016	14	1	14
10	03/06/2015	Y			07/18/2016	16	0	16
11	04/07/2015	Y			09/23/2016	18	0	18
12	04/23/2015	N	09/29/2016	17	09/29/2016	17	1	17
13	05/03/2015	Y			09/28/2016	17	0	17
14	06/18/2015	Y			09/14/2016	15	0	15
15	06/23/2015	Y			09/30/2016	15	0	15
16	07/26/2015	N	01/18/2016	6	01/18/2016	6	1	6
17	08/19/2015	Y			09/05/2016	13	0	13

(continued)

Patient Number	Enrollment Date	Alive (Y/N)	Date of Death	Time (Months) to Death	Date of Last Follow-up	Time (Months) to Last Follow-up	Event (1) or Censor (0)	Time-to-Event or Censor
18	09/23/2015	Y			09/07/2016	11	0	11
19	10/11/2015	N	08/05/2016		08/05/2016	10	1	10
20	10/15/2015	N	09/04/2016	11	09/04/2016	11	1	11
21	12/01/2015	Y			09/07/2016	9	0	9
22	01/23/2016	Y			08/31/2016	7	0	7
23	02/22/2016	Y			09/09/2016	7	0	7
24	03/03/2016	Y			08/30/2016	6	0	6
25	03/27/2016	Y			09/01/2016	5	0	5
26	04/14/2016	Y			09/19/2016	5	0	5
27	04/25/2016	N	09/19/2016	5	09/19/2016	5	1	5
28	07/17/2016	Y			09/09/2016	2	0	2
29	08/09/2016	Y			09/11/2016	1	0	1
30	08/18/2016	Y			09/20/2016	1	0	1

Note that, in the case of overall survival analysis, the time to last follow-up and time-to-event or censor columns contain the same data.

f. Median Survival ~ 22 months

g. Kaplan–Meier curve for overall survival:

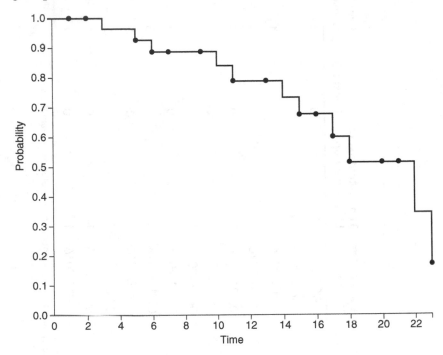

h. Log-rank test or Cox proportional hazards regression

i. Cox proportional hazards regression

2.

a. A HR of .67 means that the risk of death for those in the experimental group is only two-third of that of the standard of care group.

b. The HR of death for the standard of care group = 1/0.67 = 1.49.

c. A HR of 1.49 for the standard of care group means risk of death is 1.49 times higher in the standard of care group than in the experimental group.

3. Appropriate statistical tests:

a. Linear regression (continuous independent variable [age] and continuous dependent variable [Hgb]).

b. i. Logistic regression (no time component)

ii. Chi-square

c. Kaplan–Meier/Log-rank

d. Cox proportional hazards/Cox regression

BASICS OF EPIDEMIOLOGY

Study Designs

11

EXPERIMENTAL STUDIES

Experimental studies are central to oncology research. These prospective studies are designed to examine the effects of an intervention on a result or outcome.

CLINICAL TRIALS

Clinical trials are experimental studies conducted with human subjects. Clinical trials are always prospective. In oncology, the intervention examined is often a treatment (e.g., chemotherapeutic agent, targeted agent, radiotherapy, oncologist approach), and the outcomes of interest often include disease response, disease-free survival, overall survival, incidence of side effects, or quality of life. Clinical trials may also be developed to test two treatment strategies against one another to determine which of the two results in the best outcome.

Designing a clinical trial requires a great deal of preparation and resources. A thorough understanding of the appropriate design, analysis, and goals is critical to developing a successful clinical trial.

Unfortunately, our ability to translate basic science cancer research to successful clinical trials is very low. In fact, clinical trials in oncology have some of the highest failure rates of all clinical trials. This relative lack of success may be due, in part, to issues related to clinical trial design. This highlights the importance of appropriate clinical trial strategy. Investigators who design oncology clinical trials must have extensive knowledge of clinical statistics and an in-depth understanding of trial principles.

Common Outcomes for Clinical Trials in Oncology

Survival is a measure of the number or percentage of patients alive during a given study time period.

Mortality is a measure of the number or percentage of patients who died during a given study time period.

Incidence is a measure of the number of NEW diagnoses or cases in a dataset over the defined period of the trial. This is often the endpoint in prevention and screening trials.

Prevalence is a measure of the number or proportion of cases in a population at a given time.

Time to progression (TTP) is a measure of the time that passes between the defined start period for analysis (e.g., randomization) and the first sign of progression of cancer (e.g., new sites of disease or enlargement of known disease as measured by Response Evaluation Criteria in Solid Tumors [RECIST] criteria [1]).

Objective tumor response rate is a measure of the proportion of patients in a trial who experience a substantial reduction in the pre-study tumor burden, often measured by RECIST or other criteria.

Complete response rate is a measure of the proportion of patients in a trial who experience complete radiologic and clinic disappearance of all signs of cancer in response to treatment.

Disease-free survival (DFS) is an endpoint used in studying patients with no evidence of disease upon entering a study (e.g., those receiving adjuvant treatment after surgery). DFS is a measure of time that passes between the defined start period for analysis (e.g., randomization) until evidence of recurrence, new primary cancer, or death.

Event-free survival (EFS) is a measure of time that passes between the defined start period for analysis (e.g., randomization) until the occurrence of a pre-determined event (e.g., development of a particular side effect, disease recurrence). EFS and DFS are sometimes used interchangeably.

Progression-free survival (PFS) is a measure of time that passes between the defined start period for analysis (e.g., randomization) until evidence of disease progression or death. PFS is often preferred over TTP because TTP does not incorporate death.

Cause-specific survival (CSS) is a measure of time that passes between the defined start period for analysis (e.g., randomization) until death from the predetermined cause being investigated (e.g., death from lung cancer in a trial investigating patients with stage IV non-small cell lung carcinoma [NSCLC]).

Overall survival (OS) is a measure of time that passes between the defined start period for analysis (e.g., randomization) until death from any cause. Many consider OS to be the most reliable oncology endpoint.

Symptoms endpoint (patient-reported outcome) is a measure of the number or percentage of patients who develop new or worsening symptoms related to cancer. Such endpoints are often assessed by TTP of cancer symptoms.

There are four steps of "phases" of clinical trials:

Phase I Clinical Trials

Phase I clinical trials represent the first phase in testing treatments in humans. The goal of a Phase I clinical trial is to determine the safety of the therapy being tested. Phase I clinical trials are often used to determine the best treatment dose or best treatment method. When testing the effects of a new drug or a novel method or device for radiotherapy, Phase I clinical trials are often used to determine the *maximum-tolerated dose* (MTD) and any *dose-limiting toxicity* (DLT). MTD is the highest dose of a pharmaceutical, radioactive, or other treatment that will produce the desired effect without unacceptable toxicity levels. DLTs are adverse effects of pharmaceutical, radioactive, or other treatments severe enough that treatment cannot be escalated to a higher dose or level of treatment.

A "3+3" design is often used for first-in-human Phase I dose escalation trials. In such a design, subjects are enrolled in groups or cohorts defined by increasing doses. Typically three subjects are enrolled in a cohort. If those three subjects do not experience a DLT, the three subjects are enrolled in the next increasing dose cohort. If one subject develops a DLT at a certain dose, that particular dose cohort is opened to an additional three patients. If none of the additional three patients in the cohort develops a DLT, then three subjects are enrolled in the next increasing dose cohort. If a DLT is seen in more than 1 of 6 subjects in any cohort, then the MTD has been exceeded at that cohort. Thus, the dose is no longer escalated.

Example

Let us explore some examples:

The most obvious example and the easiest to understand is an example of a Phase I trial with a new, investigational anti-cancer drug. In recent years in oncology, there have been few advances as influential as those in immunotherapy for the treatment of melanoma. Let us use the example of the development of combination therapy with Nivolumab and Ipilimumab for metastatic melanoma (2). This Phase I trial was a dose-escalation study, as are many Phase I clinical trials testing new oncology drugs.

The initial Phase I dose escalation trial was conducted as follows:

Study Design

This Phase I study was a multi-center, multi-dose, dose escalation study of patients with unresectable stage III or stage IV melanoma comprising a total of eight dose cohorts: six concurrent regimens and two sequential regimens. The trial design was a standard 3+3 design. The investigated dose levels for each cohort were defined as follows:

Concurrent Regimens		
Cohort	Nivolumab Dose (mg/kg)	Ipilimumab Dose (mg/kg)
1	0.3	3
2	1	3
2a	3	1
3	3	3
4	10	3
5	10	10

Sequenced Regimens		
Cohort	Nivolumab Dose (mg/kg)	Ipilimumab Dose (mg/kg)
6	1	Prior
7	3	Prior

Primary Endpoint

The primary endpoint in this study was defined as the safety and tolerability of the combination treatment. The severity of adverse events was graded according to the National Cancer Institute Common Terminology Criteria for Adverse Events, version 3.0. DLT was defined as a toxicity requiring discontinuation of the study drug. All Grade 5 toxicity, any Grade 4 nonhematologic toxicity (with the exception of lymphopenia, neutropenia lasting less than or equal to 48 hours and not associated with fever or clinical symptoms, or certain Grade 4 electrolyte abnormalities) or any Grade 4 nonhematologic toxicity were considered DLTs.

Sample Size

A total of 86 patients were treated in the study. For the concurrent regimen cohorts, the trial design was initially that three patients would be treated at each dose level if no dose limiting toxicity were noted. If this was the case, the next three patients would be treated in the subsequent cohort at the next dose level. If DLT was noted, three additional patients would be treated in the cohort at the dose at which the toxicity occurred. If those three patients did not experience DLT, the patients enrolled next would be treated in the subsequent cohort at the next dose level. This Phase I protocol also incorporated a cohort expansion to a total of up to 16 patients at the maximum doses that were associated with an acceptable level of adverse events or the maximum administered dose.

The study design called for approximately 96 subjects to be enrolled based on the following calculations:

"If among 12 subjects at each dose there are 1 (8.3%), 2 (17%), or 3 (25%) events of interest observed, then the 70% confidence interval for this event rate would be (1.4%, 25%), (5.8%, 35%), or (11.4%, 44%) respectively, or equivalently there is 85% confidence that the event rate observed in similar future trials would not be higher than 25%, 35%, or 44%, respectively. In addition, with 16 subjects at the MTD or similar dose, the 70% confidence interval for a tumor response rate would be (4.3% to 27%) if 2 (12.5%) subjects had a tumor response, and it would be (8.5% to 34%) if 3 (19%) subjects had a tumor response."

Evaluation

The period for evaluating DLT for the purposes of dose escalation was nine weeks. If no subject in a dose cohort experienced DLT within nine weeks, then the study moved to enroll the next three subjects at the next dose cohort level. If one subject of the initial three in any dose cohort experienced DLT within the nine-week interval, the cohort was planned to be expanded to six subjects. If the remainder of those six subjects experienced no DLT within nine weeks, the study was planned to move to enroll the next three subjects at the next dose cohort level. However, if any additional patients within a cohort (beyond the first one of the six subjects to experience DLT) experienced DLT, the cohort was planned to be defined as having exceeded the MTD. All subjects were observed for toxicity in the clinic during each infusion and for at least two hours afterward. Additional visits for safety were scheduled every six weeks from week 42 to week 102 and at week 30.

Results

Dose cohort three was found to exceed the MTD (Nivolumab at a dose of three mg per kilogram and Ipilimumab at a dose of three mg per kilogram) as three of the six patients had G3 toxicity that persisted for greater than or equal to three weeks. The doses in cohort two (Nivolumab at one mg per kilogram and Ipilimumab at three mg per kilogram) were considered MTD as they were associated with an acceptable level of adverse events.

Example

It may also be helpful to look at an example of a Phase I clinical trial in radiation oncology. Using the well-known example of the development of stereotactic body radiotherapy (SBRT) for treatment of early-stage lung tumors in patients considered medically inoperable, we see that Phase I clinical trials in radiotherapy are often dose-finding studies (3,4).

The initial Phase I dose escalation trial was conducted as follows:

Study Design

This Phase I study was a dose escalation study investigating the safety of SBRT in patients with medically inoperable stage I primary NSCLC. An initial SBRT dose level of 24 Gy in three fractions was chosen. The dose was escalated by six Gy (two Gy per fraction) until MTD was reached. When the 42 Gy dose level was reached, separate dose escalations were carried out for patients with T1 tumors ($\leq$3 cm) and T2 tumors ($\leq$7 cm) for that and each subsequent dose level. This study had a standard 3+3 design.

Primary Endpoint

The primary endpoint was defined as a tumoricidal dose at or approaching the MTD for the eligible patients. DLT was defined as any Grade 3 pulmonary, esophageal, cardiac, or pericardial toxicity, or any Grade 4 toxicity that was ascribed to the protocol treatment.

Sample Size

A minimum of three patients were treated at each dose level. If only one patient in a dose cohort experienced DLT, an additional two patients would be accrued at that dose level. If no additional DLT was noted in these two patients, dose escalation to the next dose level would proceed. If any of the additional two patients experienced DLT, MTD would have been exceeded. Overall, if two or more of the patients treated at a given dose level experienced DLT, MTD would have been exceeded. A total of 37 patients were treated in the study.

Evaluation

A minimum observation period for toxicity was defined in the trial as follows: If the first patient in each dose cohort did not experience DLT, the second patient was followed for a minimum of four weeks without DLT before the third patient could be enrolled. The third patient was followed for a minimum of two weeks without DLT before the next cohort was initiated.

Results

For T1 tumors, MTD was not achieved. For T2 tumors larger than five cm in size, DLT was observed at the 72 Gy dose with three out of five patients experiencing Grade 3 or higher toxicity. As such, MTD for this tumor subset was defined at 66 Gy.

Phase II Clinical Trials

In the next step or phase of clinical trials, Phase II, the goal is an initial assessment of efficacy of clinical activity. Essentially, the goal of Phase II trials is to screen out ineffective drugs and to identify promising new drugs for Phase III evaluation. Phase II trials also serve to further define safety and toxicity of the treatments beyond what was seen in Phase I trials.

Phase II trials are often developed to assess response to investigational new drugs for a particular disease. Alternatively, a Phase II trial may be developed to further assess previously tested treatments with regards to a new treatment schedule, a new disease, or use of the drug in combination with another drug.

The most simple and easy-to-understand example of a Phase II trial is a single-arm efficacy trial of a novel oncologic agent. In oncology, this type of trial comprises administering a drug and assessing response. Response may be coded as a binary categorical dependent variable (i.e., there is either a clinical response or no clinical response). More complicated Phase II trials look at overall survival or time-to-event data. Traditional Phase II trials are single-arm studies. In order to determine efficacy, the results of single-arm Phase II trials are often compared with the results from historical controls. Such a method predisposes to bias and confounding. This could be particularly problematic when comparing time-to-event data such as survival that changes over time due to medical advances unrelated to cancer treatment. As a result, simple single-arm Phase II trials are at risk for Type I error.

What about randomized Phase II trials? Randomized Phase II trials compare two contemporary groups. The randomization is often between an experimental treatment and the standard of care. Alternatively, the randomization may be between two experimental groups. The goal of randomized Phase II trials might be to determine whether a particular experimental regimen should be brought forward for further testing. Common endpoints include objective tumor response rate, complete response rate, PFS, or OS. Following a Phase II trial, a subsequent trial would commonly be a randomized Phase III trial designed to compare the experimental regimen to a standard regimen, often with overall survival as an endpoint (see the section Phase III Clinical Trials).

Example

Following the publication of the Phase I trial of combined Ipilimumab and Nivolumab in metastatic melanoma (2), a Phase II trial examining combination Ipilimumab and Nivolumab was published (5).

This randomized Phase II trial was conducted as follows:

Study Design

This Phase II double-blind, randomized trial randomized patients with previously untreated stage III or IV melanoma with measurable disease in a 2:1 fashion to either standard of care (Ipilimumab) plus placebo every three weeks for four doses followed by placebo every two weeks or to experimental treatment (Ipilimumab plus Nivolumab) every three weeks for four doses followed by maintenance Nivolumab every two weeks. The statistical null hypothesis (H_0) stated that there was no difference in objective response rate in patients receiving Ipilimumab plus placebo versus in patients receiving Ipilimumab plus Nivolumab.

Primary Endpoint

The primary endpoint was the investigator-assessed objective response rate (ORR) among patients with BRAF v600E wild-type tumors.

Sample Size

A total of 142 patients were included in the study. The following calculations were used to estimate a treatment goal of 100 subjects. Preliminary data revealed an expected ORR of approximately 50%. With an observed ORR close to this expected ORR, a 95% confidence interval (CI) would be approximately 40% to 60%. With 100 subjects, an observed ORR of 50% would support that the true ORR is greater than or equal to approximately 40% with a Type I error rate of 5%.

Results

The results revealed confirmed ORR of 61% in the experimental group and 11% in the group that received standard of care plus placebo. The *p*-value for this comparison was .0001, and as such, the null hypothesis was rejected. The hazard ratio associated with combination therapy as compared with Ipilimumab monotherapy for disease progression or death (endpoint of PFS) was .40 with a 95% CI of .23 to .68.

Example

For the radiation oncologists, let us continue with the example of the development of SBRT as treatment for early-stage NSCLC in patients considered medically inoperable. Following the Phase I trial detailed earlier, a single-arm Phase II trial of SBRT in the treatment of patients with medically inoperable stage I NSCLC, RTOG 0236, was developed and conducted (6,7).

Study Design

This single-arm prospective Phase II trial of SBRT was conducted in patients with medically inoperable stage T1 or T2 (with tumors measuring ≤ 7 cm) NSCLC. Patients were treated with SBRT to 60 to 66 Gy and followed.

Primary Endpoint

The primary endpoint was two-year actuarial primary tumor control defined as the absence of local growth.

Sample Size

A total of 59 patients were enrolled, and 55 were evaluable. The sample size was determined from the Phase II trial's goal to improve upon the historical two-year control rate of 60% to 80%. The trial assumed an approximately exponential distribution of time to local progression and calculated the hazard rate for a local control of 80% and 60% to be .0093 and .02128 per month, respectively. It was calculated that 18 cases of local progression were required for a Type I error rate of .05% with 80% power to detect a difference. Based on this calculation, a total of 49 patients accrued over just over two years were needed. With a 5% rate of ineligibility or inevaluability, it was determined that 52 patients were required for this trial.

Evaluation

Final analysis was planned after each patient had a minimum of 24 months of follow-up. Interim reports were prepared every six months, including accrual rates, patient characteristics, and the frequency and severity of toxicities.

Results

Long-term results were presented at the American Society for Radiation Oncology (ASTRO) 2014 annual meeting with four years median follow-up and the estimated five-year primary tumor failure rate was 7%.

Example

More recently, with publications including the I-SPY 2 trial in breast cancer, researchers have incorporated Bayesian interim monitoring into Phase II clinical trials (8,9). Bayesian analysis, you may remember from medical school, depends on a pretest probability. Bayesian analysis is very different from standard analysis. There are no CIs or *p*-values, and data can be analyzed at any time. The Bayesian interim monitoring is an adaptive strategy that matches therapies with the patients most likely to benefit from such therapies.

The Bayesian method used in the I-SPY 2 trial follows three steps that are repeated throughout the course of the study: (a) start, (b) observe, and (c) combine. The technique starts by defining a hypothesis and an associated prediction at the start of the experiment before there is any true data. Next, the data obtained is observed and used to determine the true likelihood of an effect. Finally, the prediction and the observed data are combined to re-estimate the distribution of the effect. A predictive probability is calculated from this distribution, and the higher the Bayesian probability (the closer to 1), the better the chance of concluding a positive result.

The I-SPY 2 trial sought to compare up to 12 experimental therapies with a common control in subgroups of breast cancer with 10 distinct biomarker signatures. The randomization was stratified across the biomarker subgroups. Throughout the course of the trial, randomization was adaptive such that patients within each strata were randomized to receive agents that were more likely to be efficacious based on the previous data. Thus far, two therapies (Neratinib in Her2+, Hormone Receptor–negative breast cancer and combination Veliparib–Carboplatin in triple-negative breast cancer) have met pre-specified criteria for testing in larger Phase III trials.

Phase III Clinical Trials

The goal of a Phase III clinical trial is to definitively test the efficacy of a drug or other treatment for a particular condition. The ideal Phase III clinical trial is a randomized, double-blind, placebo-controlled clinical trial comparing the current standard of care to a new therapy that has been successful in both Phase I and Phase II trials.

Example

In fact, only approximately one-third of the therapies progress past Phase II trials to Phase III trials. The combination therapy of Nivolumab plus Ipilimumab is an example of one such therapy. The CheckMate 067 study, published in the *New England Journal of Medicine* in 2016 and presented at the American Society for Clinical Oncology (ASCO) 2016 annual meeting, is a randomized, double-blind Phase III trial investigating this combination in unresectable or metastatic melanoma (10,11).

The Phase III study was conducted as follows:

Study Design

In this randomized, double-blind, Phase III study trial, treatment-naïve patients with unresectable stage III or stage IV melanoma were randomly assigned, in parallel, without the knowledge of the patient or the investigator, to one of the three arms:

A. An experimental arm that included Nivolumab and placebo for Ipilimumab

B. An experimental arm that included Nivolumab and Ipilimumab

C. A standard of care arm that included Ipilimumab and placebo for Nivolumab

In each arm, therapy was delivered until documented disease progression, discontinuation due to toxicity, withdrawal of consent, or the study ended.

Primary Endpoints

The co-primary endpoints were defined as OS and PFS.

Sample Size

As of the publication in the *New England Journal of Medicine* in 2015, 1296 patients were enrolled and 945 patients underwent randomization. Sample size calculations estimated enrollment at 915 patients. In designing the study, investigators determined that at least 460 events would be needed in each OS comparison to provide at least 90% power to detect a hazard ratio of .72 (which corresponds to a 39% increase in median OS assuming a median overall survival of 14 months for Ipilimumab and 19.4 months for each of the experimental groups) with a Type I error rate of .025 (two-sided).

Evaluation

Patients were assessed for tumor response according to RECIST criteria beginning 12 weeks after randomization, then every six weeks for 49 weeks, and then every 12 weeks until progression or treatment discontinuation.

Results

The first results of this trial were presented in a peer-reviewed publication in the *New England Journal of Medicine* in 2015, and in abstract form as an oral presentation at the 2016 ASCO meeting. Median follow-up was 20.7 months. Median PFS was 11.5 months for those treated with combination Nivolumab and Ipilimumab as compared to 6.9 months for those treated with Nivolumab alone and 2.9 months for those treated with Ipilimumab alone.

Phase IV Clinical Trials

Phase IV trials are conducted after a therapy has been licensed. The goal of a Phase IV trial is to gather additional information about the efficacy and long-term toxicity of a therapy.

Example

Combination therapy with Nivolumab and Ipilimumab is pending Phase IV trials; however, there is an ongoing national Phase IV study with Ipilimumab for patients with advanced melanoma run by the Oslo University Hospital (https://clinicaltrials.gov/ct2/show/NCT02068196). The authors state that the goal of the study is to "understand how Ipilimumab is being used, its safety profile, and the manner in which adverse reactions are managed in routine clinical practice."

This Phase IV study is ongoing and was/is conducted as follows:

Study Design

Patients with biopsy confirmed unresectable stage III or stage IV melanoma treated with Ipilimumab are observed and data is to be collected with respect the primary, secondary, and additional endpoints between enrollment after January 2014 and December 2018.

Primary Endpoints

The primary endpoint of this Phase IV trial is to determine the number of patients receiving Ipilimumab who develop serious and nonserious adverse reactions.

Sample Size

The estimated enrollment is 150 patients.

Evaluation

Patients were/are evaluated for toxicity, progression, and survival at regular intervals before each Ipilimumab dose and every 12 weeks until progression or up to five years. Quality of life assessment was/is obtained before each Ipilimumab dose and every 12 weeks until progression. Serum and plasma biomarkers, SNP, RNA, and immunological response analysis were/are performed before weeks one, four, and seven and before months three, six, 12, 24, and 36.

Results

Not yet presented.

Meta-Analysis

A meta-analysis is a statistical analysis that combines the qualitative and quantitative study data of multiple scientific studies or clinical trials that address a similar clinical question. The statistical analysis yields a weighted average from the results of individual studies. Aggregation of information from multiple smaller studies into one large meta-analysis allows for increased statistical power to detect the effect being examined. A meta-analysis also includes a sample with overall greater diversity among subjects.

Clinical trials in oncology, particularly clinical trials in the United States, are often limited by accrual such that estimated enrollment is not always achieved. Moreover, in the case that estimated enrollment is reached, power could still be improved upon or a more accurate estimate of effect size could be achieved by combining samples from multiple separate clinical trials. In a situation where multiple clinical trials testing the same treatment or intervention achieve conflicting results, a meta-analysis could be designed to clarify the overall results.

A meta-analysis is a type of systemic review, and all meta-analyses must begin with a carefully conducted systemic review. When a question appropriate for meta-analysis is identified, all the related published and unpublished studies should be evaluated. Scientific, clinical, and statistical judgment should be used to determine which of these published and unpublished studies is appropriate for inclusion in the analysis. Meta-analysis requires sophisticated statistical techniques.

The Early Breast Cancer Trialists' Collaborative Group (EBCTCG) has undertaken multiple meta-analyses of clinical trials in breast cancer. An excellent example is a meta-analysis of randomized trials comparing aromatase inhibitors versus tamoxifen in the treatment of early breast cancer (12).

The meta-analysis was conducted as follows:

Study Design

A total of nine eligible clinical trials comparing aromatase inhibitors versus tamoxifen in women with estrogen receptor-positive (ER-positive) early-stage breast cancer were included in this meta-analysis. All included trials were conducted beginning by 2005. Individual patient datasets for 31,920 randomized patients were analyzed. Log-rank statistics were used to assess the effect of aromatase inhibitors versus tamoxifen on various outcomes.

Primary Outcomes

The primary outcomes of the meta-analysis were any recurrence of breast cancer, breast cancer mortality, death without recurrence, and all-cause mortality.

Evaluation

Information regarding patient and tumor characteristics, as well as dates of any breast cancer recurrence, additional primary cancer, bone fractures, death, and cause of death were sought between 2012 and 2014.

Results

Ten-year recurrence risk was 19.1% in the aromatase inhibitor group versus 22.7% in the tamoxifen group; a statistically significant difference ($p < .00001$). Ten-year breast cancer mortality was statistically significantly lower with aromatase inhibitors than with tamoxifen (12.1% vs. 14.2%, $p = .009$).

FIELD TRIALS

Field trials are different from clinical trials, in that they are generally performed in a healthy population as opposed to being performed on patients. Field trials are typically prophylactic and focused on prevention, as opposed to clinical trials, which are typically therapeutic and are focused on treatment.

COMMUNITY INTERVENTION TRIALS

Community intervention trials are epidemiologic studies. Intervention trials may be conducted with the intention of reducing risk for or treating a disease such as cancer.

The Community Intervention Trial for Smoking Cessation (COMMIT) is an example of a community intervention trial in oncology conducted from 1989 to 1991. This multi-center project was established with the goal of putting forth a community-wide smoking cessation program.

Study Design

Eleven matched pairs of communities, including 10,019 heavy smokers and 10,328 light-to-moderate smokers were studied. One community in each pair underwent interventions to promote smoking cessation using community resources and the other community in each pair acted as a control.

Data Analysis

Smoking quit rates were compared among those communities that underwent intervention and those communities that did not.

Results

The light-to-moderate smoker quit rates were statistically significantly higher in smokers in the intervention communities than those in the control communities (.306 vs. .275; $p = .047$) (13).

NONEXPERIMENTAL STUDIES

COHORT STUDIES

A cohort study is a longitudinal study developed to answer a clinical question. In a cohort study, patients are divided into two groups, or cohorts, based on the presence or absence of a certain risk factor or intervention during a certain period. The two groups are then compared with respect to incidence of a particular outcome. Cohort studies can be carried out in a retrospective or prospective fashion.

RETROSPECTIVE COHORT STUDY

Example

A simple example of a retrospective cohort study examining the relationship between vasectomy and prostate cancer was published in the *Journal of the American Medical Association (JAMA)* in 1993 (14).

Study Design

In this retrospective cohort study, 14,607 women in the Nurses' Health Study whose partners had had vasectomy were compared to 14,607 age-matched women in the same study whose partners had not had a vasectomy. In total, 26,103 of these women were contacted retrospectively to determine whether their partners had developed prostate cancer.

Data Analysis

Analysis of the data was based upon yearly incidence of prostate cancer. The Cox proportional hazards model was used to assess the relative risk of developing prostate cancer while accounting for time-dependent covariates.

Results

During the study, 96 new cases of prostate cancer were diagnosed; 37 cases developed in men who had no vasectomy and 59 in men who had vasectomy.

Vasectomy was associated with an increased risk of prostate cancer with an age-adjusted relative risk of 1.56 and a p-value of .04. With increased time since vasectomy, the number of new cases of prostate cancer per year increased.

PROSPECTIVE COHORT STUDY

Example

In the same issue of *JAMA*, the same authors published a prospective cohort study examining the relationship between vasectomy and prostate cancer (15).

Study Design

This prospective cohort study included 10,055 male health professions between the ages of 40 and 75 years who had previously had a vasectomy and 37,800 male health professionals between the same ages who had not had a vasectomy.

Data Analysis

Very similar to the retrospective version of this study detailed earlier, the primary analysis was based on yearly incidence rates within the cohort. Vasectomy was first dichotomized and then categorized into time to vasectomy. Censoring occurred at diagnosis of prostate cancer, death, or end-of-study period. The relative risk was computed as the rate of prostate cancer diagnosis among men with vasectomy divided by the rate of prostate cancer diagnosis among men who had not had vasectomy. The Mantel–Haenszel test was used to adjust for covariates.

Results

During the study, 300 new cases of prostate cancer and 279 cases of greater than A1 prostate cancer were diagnosed; 225 of the 37,800 men who had no vasectomy, and 54 of the 1,055 men who had vasectomy were diagnosed with prostate cancer greater than A1. Vasectomy was associated with an increased risk of prostate cancer with an age-adjusted relative risk for vasectomy of 1.66 and a p-value of .0004.

CASE-CONTROL STUDIES

Case-control studies retrospectively compare groups of subjects based on the outcome. To carry out a case-control study, investigators must start with the outcome—typically the presence of a diagnosis such as cancer. The group of cases comprises those with the outcome in question (e.g., cancer) and the group of controls comprises those without the outcome in question (e.g., no cancer). The two groups are then retrospectively compared to identify any risk factors that differ between the two groups.

Example

An example of a case-control study of human papillomavirus (HPV) and oropharyngeal cancer was published in the *New England Journal of Medicine* in 2007 (16).

Study Design

This retrospective case-control study identified patients based on the presence or absence of oropharyngeal cancer. The investigators identified 100 patients with newly diagnosed oropharyngeal cancer (case patients) and compared them to 200 patients without cancer (control patients).

Data Analysis

The two groups were compared with regard to HPV infection status using multivariable logistic regression models. Odds ratios were calculated for each comparison and adjusted for age, sex, tobacco use, alcohol use, dentition and tooth brushing, and the presence or absence of a family history of head and neck cancer. Totally, 95% CIs were calculated for each odds ratio. Multivariate models were created through a step-wise approach, whereby variables that were not significant in the univariate analysis were eliminated and those deemed biologically relevant were retained.

Results

Oropharyngeal cancer was strongly associated with serologic measures of exposure to HPV-16 and with the presence of oral HPV infection. A total of 57 (57%) of the case patients and 14 (7%) of control patients were seropositive for HPV-16 L1, with an odds ratio of 17.6 and an adjusted odds ratio of 32.2. Oral HPV infection was found in 32 (32%) of cases and eight (4%) of the control patients with an odds ratio of 11.3 and an adjusted odds ratio of 14.6.

COHORT STUDIES VERSUS CASE-CONTROL STUDIES

To answer the question "Is smoking associated with risk of lung cancer?," let us describe the design of (a) a retrospective cohort study, (b) a prospective cohort study, and (c) a case-control study that would appropriately examine the clinical question.

- *Retrospective cohort study*: Identify a cohort of patients who smoke and a cohort of patients with no smoking history. Examine each patient's medical history to determine how many smokers have developed lung cancer compared to how many never-smokers have developed lung cancer. Retrospectively compare the lung cancer incidence between the two groups.

- *Prospective cohort study*: Identify a cohort of patients who smoke and a cohort of patients with no smoking history. Follow each patient for 10 years to determine how many smokers develop lung cancer compared to how many never-smokers develop lung cancer during that 10-year time period. After 10 years, compare the lung cancer incidence between the two groups.

- *Case-control study*: Identify a group of patients with lung cancer (cases) and a group of patient without lung cancer (controls) to be included in the study. Compare the two groups retrospectively to see whether they differ as to the percentage of smokers in each group.

CROSS-SECTIONAL STUDIES

Cross-sectional studies gather data from a population sample at a single time point from groups that differ with respect to a variable of interest, but are otherwise similar. Observations from each group at a specific point in time are compared. There is no intervention and no manipulation by the researchers. Cross-sectional studies are information gathering studies only.

Example

An example of a cross-sectional study examining psychological distress in cancer patients during chemotherapy was presented at the 2016 Palliative and Supportive Care in Oncology Symposium (17). Responses from the Depression, Anxiety, Stress Scale 21 (DASS 21) were obtained from 300 cancer patients and 300 controls in the state of Punjab, India, at a point in time. There was no intervention. The observations included the responses on the DASS 21. The results revealed a statistically significant difference in mean DASS 21 scores between cancer patients and controls.

MATCHED STUDIES

Matched studies are designed such that subjects within each group to be studied are matched in pairs. Outcomes are compared within each matched pair. A matched pair design is intended to control for potential confounders in the variables that are being matched.

Example

A matched pair analysis comparing surgery followed by radiotherapy versus radiotherapy alone for metastatic spinal cord compression was published in the *Journal of Clinical Oncology* in 2010 (18).

Study Design

In this study, 108 patients who underwent surgery plus radiotherapy for malignant spinal cord compression were matched 1:2 to 216 controls who were treated with radiotherapy alone based on 11 potential prognostic factors, including age, gender, Eastern Cooperative Oncology Group (ECOG) performance status (PS), type of primary tumor, number of involved vertebrae, other bone metastases, visceral metastases, interval from tumor diagnosis to malignant spinal cord compression, ambulatory status before treatment, time developing motor deficits before treatment, and radiotherapy regimen.

Primary Endpoint

The primary endpoint was the post-treatment ambulatory rate.

Data Analysis

To account for the matched-pair design, a stratified Cox regression model with backward selection of variables was used.

Results

There was no significant difference in the post-treatment ambulatory rate between those undergoing surgery followed by radiotherapy and those undergoing radiotherapy alone.

ANALYSIS OF STUDIES

CRUDE ANALYSIS

Relative risks, odds ratios, and hazard ratios are crude estimators of effect size in different types of experimental studies and clinical trials. The crude approximations represented by these estimators may be modified by bias, confounding, and effect modification, as follows.

BIAS

Bias refers to systematic error in experimental design that leads to an inaccurate estimate of the effect size, and as a result, to inaccurate conclusions of a study. In biostatistical studies, bias is most often due to selection or measurement bias.

Selection bias is the result of selection of subjects who have characteristics different from the characteristics of the population the subject sample was intended to represent.

Example

For example, think of a cross-sectional study evaluating the relationship between socioeconomic status and financial loss during cancer treatment. Imagine the study is conducted at a large public academic cancer center known to serve a large proportion of uninsured patients. Prior research has shown that the average income of patients treated at the cancer center is lower than the average income of residents in the city in which the cancer center is located and lower than the average income in the United States. Thus, selection bias exists, in that patients included in the study are not necessarily representative of the regional or national population of patients undergoing cancer treatment.

Randomization and matching are two methods often used to reduce selection bias.

Measurement bias is the result of use of an imperfect risk classification system or an inaccurate measure of outcomes in a study design. An example of an imperfect risk classification could occur when subjects in a study are categorized based on their responses to a survey or questionnaire. Inaccurate measure of outcomes may be due to either observer or responder bias.

Example

Let us again imagine a cross-sectional study evaluating socioeconomic status and financial loss during cancer treatment. Subjects are mailed a questionnaire with questions regarding their socioeconomic status prior to a cancer diagnosis. Measurement bias may occur if patients are not truthful in answering the questionnaire for any reason (e.g., lack of knowledge of their true financial standings or a desire to be perceived as having more or less wealth than they actually have). Incorrect survey answers will lead to incorrect assessment of socioeconomic status and bias of study results. This is an example of measurement bias due to responder bias.

Investigator and subject blinding are methods often used to reduce measurement bias.

CONFOUNDING

Confounding refers to undue influence on study results by a variable (a variable that is not accounted for) other than the independent/risk variable. A confounding variable is a variable that is related to the defined independent/risk variable and is separately associated with the outcome/dependent variable.

Example

Let us again use the preceding example of a cross-sectional study evaluating the relationship between socioeconomic status and financial loss during cancer treatment conducted at a large public academic cancer center known to serve a large proportion of uninsured low-income patients. We can imagine that overall prognosis may be a potential confounder. Low socioeconomic status has been associated with inferior cancer outcomes. Overall cancer prognosis has an obvious influence on a patient's ability to earn during and after treatment. Thus, cancer prognosis meets the definition of a confounder, in that it is related to the risk variable socioeconomic status and is independently associated with financial loss related to cancer treatment.

STRATIFIED ANALYSIS

Stratification is a method to address confounding in studies and clinical trials. This method is appropriate when confounding variables are known at the time of study design. With stratification, subjects in the study are analyzed separately based on the status of the confounder.

Example

A recent randomized, international, open-label Phase III trial published in the *New England Journal of Medicine* compared PFS for patients with EGFRT790M–positive lung cancer who received treatment with osimertinib to PFS for those who received platinum-pemetrexed chemotherapy (19). In designing this Phase III trial, the investigators acknowledged race (Asian vs. non-Asian) as a potential confounding factor. To account for this, patients in the trial were stratified according to Asian or non-Asian race before randomization. Analysis of PFS using the log-rank test was stratified according to Asian or non-Asian race.

EFFECT MODIFICATION

Effect medication occurs if an effect that truly exists is observed in a study or trial, but the magnitude of that effect is altered (either strengthened or weakened) by an associated variable.

Example

Age and gender are examples of variables that often result in effect modification. As an example, consider the effect of age on prognosis in head and neck cancer. The meta analysis of chemotherapy in head and neck cancer (MACH-NC) comparing trials of locoregional treatment alone against trials of locoregional treatment combined with chemotherapy in patients with squamous cell carcinoma of the head and neck demonstrated effect modification based on age (20). The log-rank test was used to compare OS between the groups and hazard ratios for death were calculated. Overall, the hazard ratio (HR) of death was .88 ($p < .0001$) with an absolute benefit for chemotherapy of 4.5% at five years. To study the effect modification of age (as a covariate) on treatment, an analysis stratified by trial was performed, and the hazard ratio for age was compared by a test for trend. There was a decreasing beneficial effect of chemotherapy with increasing age. According to the authors, this effect could not be explained by an imbalance in the other covariates studied. In this meta-analysis, the effect of the addition of chemotherapy to locoregional treatment on reducing the HR for death to .88 was likely weakened by the effect of age and by the inclusion of elderly patients.

CONNECTIONS TO REGRESSIONS

Regressions are often incorporated in clinical trials, meta-analyses, cohort studies, case-control studies, and cross-sectional studies. Regressions in clinical trials are used to adjust for prognostic variables to allow for better estimates of the treatment effect. The effect of regression in clinical trials is to reduce variability between subjects to allow for increased power and more narrow CIs.

Let us review the type of regression appropriate for each type of study and clinical trial.

A Cox Proportional Hazards Regression (see Chapter 8, section titled Cox Proportional Hazards Model) is used to evaluate the effect of multiple variables, known as covariates, on a time-to-event outcome (e.g., PFS, OS).

A simple linear regression (see Chapter 6, section titled Simple Linear Regression) is used to evaluate the singular effect of one independent variable on a continuous dependent variable. A simple linear regression could be used in a cross-sectional or cohort study with a continuous outcome variable that does not have a time-to event-component. In many biostatistical and oncologic studies, a simple linear regression is referred to as a "univariable" analysis.

A multiple linear regression (see Chapter 6, section titled Multiple Linear Regression) is used to evaluate the effects of multiple independent variables on a continuous dependent variable. A multiple linear regression could be used in a cross-sectional or cohort study with a continuous outcome variable that does not have a time-to-event component. In many biostatistical and oncologic studies, a multiple linear regression is referred to as a "multivariable" analysis.

A simple logistic regression (see Chapter 6, section titled Logistic Regression) is used to evaluate the singular effect of one independent variable on a categorical dependent variable. A simple logistic regression could be used in a cross-sectional, cohort study, or case-control study with a categorical outcome variable that does not have a time-to event-component. In many biostatistical and oncologic studies, a simple logistic regression is referred to as a "univariable" analysis.

A multiple logistic regression (see Chapter 6, section titled Logistic Regression) is used to evaluate the effects of multiple independent variables on a categorical dependent variable. A multiple logistic regression could be used in a cross-sectional, cohort study, or case-control study with a categorical outcome variable that does not have a time-to event-component. In many biostatistical and oncologic studies, a multiple logistic regression is referred to as a "multivariable" analysis.

For analysis of time-to-event data, the log-rank test is typically used for univariable analysis and Cox proportional hazards/regression is used for multivariable analysis.

The terms "univariate" and "multivariate" analysis are very often used in oncology literature when describing univariable or multivariable analyses, respectively. This is very confusing for those of us trying to conduct, write, read, or interpret papers using these terms. For the purposes of this text, we will acknowledge that the terms "univariable" and "univariate" and typically used interchangeably in the literature. The terms "multivariable" and "multivariate" are typically used interchangeably in the literature.

SAMPLE SIZE

HYPOTHESIS TESTING

A clinical trial must enroll a minimum number of patients in order to allow for a reasonable likelihood that the desired effect will be seen if the effect, in reality, does exist. Such sample size requirements are heavily dependent upon alpha and beta.

t-Test

To calculate the minimum sample size for a *t*-test, you must define alpha and beta, and you must have an estimate of the proportion of subjects in each group (for example, if you expect half of the subjects to come from each group, the proportion of subjects would be .5 for each group), an estimate of the expected effect size, and an estimate of the standard deviation of the outcome of the population.

Testing Binomial Proportions

To calculate the minimum sample size for a test of binomial proportions, you must define alpha and beta, and you must have an estimate of the proportion of subjects in each group, an estimate of the baseline risk, and an estimate of the projected risk, the odds ratio, or the risk ratio.

Survival Analysis

To calculate the minimum sample size for a survival analysis, you must define alpha and beta, and you must have an estimate of the proportion of subjects in each group and an estimate of the approximated relative hazard ratio for the event.

Regression Analysis

For a given clinical trial, analysis by regression requires a particular sample size dependent upon the number of variables being investigated in the regression. For a multiple linear regression, the sample size should accommodate at least 10 observations (10 patients experiencing an event) for each variable. For a logistic regression, the sample size should accommodate at least 10 observations, with each of the possible dichotomous outcomes for each variable.

REFERENCES

1. Therasse P, Arbuck SG, Eisenhauer EA, et al. New guidelines to evaluate response to treatment in solid tumors. European Organization for Research and Treatment of Cancer, National Cancer Institute of the United States, National Cancer Institute of Canada. *J Natl Cancer Inst.* 2000;92:205–216. doi:10.1093/jnci/92.3.205
2. Wolchok JD, Kluger H, Callahan MK, et al. Nivolumab plus ipilimumab in advanced melanoma. *N Engl J Med.* 2013;369:122–133. doi:10.1056/NEJMoa1302369
3. Timmerman R, Papiez L, McGarry R, et al. Extracranial stereotactic radioablation. *Chest.* 2003;124:1946–1955. doi:10.1378/chest.124.5.1946
4. McGarry RC, Papiez L, Williams M, et al. Stereotactic body radiation therapy for early-stage non-small-cell lung carcinoma: phase I study.

Int J Radiation Oncology Biol Phys. 2005;63:1010–1015. doi:10.1016/j. ijrobp.2005.03.073

5. Postow MA, Chesney J, Pavlick AC, et al. Nivolumab and ipilimumab vs. ipilimumab in untreated melanoma. *N Engl J Med.* 2015;372:2006–2017. doi:10.1056/NEJMoa1414428

6. Fakiris AJ, McGarry RC, Yiannoutsos CT, et al. Stereotactic body radiation therapy for early-stage non–small-cell lung carcinoma: four-year results of a prospective phase II study. *Int J Radiation Oncology Biol Phys.* 2009;75:677–682. doi:10.1016/j.ijrobp.2008.11.042

7. Timmerman RD, Hu C, Michalski J, et al. Long-term results of RTOG 0236: a phase II trial of stereotactic body radiation therapy (SBRT) in the treatment of patients with medically inoperable stage I non-small cell lung cancer. *Int J Radiation Oncology Biol Phys.* 2014;90(1 Suppl):S30. doi:10.1016/j.ijrobp.2014.05.135

8. Park JW, Liu MC, Yee D, et al. Adaptive randomization of neritinib in early breast cancer. *N Engl J Med.* 2016;375:11–22. doi:10.1056/ NEJMoa1513750

9. Rugo HS, Olopade OI, DeMichele A, et al. Adaptive randomization of veliparib–carboplatin treatment in breast cancer. *N Engl J Med.* 2016;375:23–34. doi:10.1056/NEJMoa1513749

10. Larkin J, Chiarion-Sileni V, Gonzalez R, et al. Combined nivolumab and ipilimumab or monotherapy in untreated melanoma. *N Eng J Med.* 2015;373:23–24. doi:10.1056/NEJMoa1504030

11. Wolchok JD, Chiarion-Sileni V, Gonzalez R, et al. Updated results from a phase III trial of nivolumab (NIVO) combined with ipilimumab (IPI) in treatment-naïve patients (pts) with advanced melanoma (MEL) (CheckMate 067). *J Clin Oncol.* 2016;34(15 Suppl):9505.

12. Early Breast Cancer Trialists' Collaborative Group. Aromatase inhibitors versus tamoxifen in early breast cancer: patient-level meta-analysis of the randomized trials. *Lancet.* 2015;386:1341–1352. doi:10.1016/ S0140-6736(15)61074-1

13. The COMMIT Research Group. Community intervention trial for smoking cessation (COMMIT): I. Cohort results from a four-year community intervention. *Am J Public Health.* 1995;85:183–192. doi:10.2105/ AJPH.85.2.183

14. Giovannucci E, Tosteson TD, Speizer FE, et al. A retrospective cohort study of vasectomy and prostate cancer in US men. *JAMA.* 1993;269:878–882. doi:10.1001/jama.1993.03500070058029

15. Giovannucci E, Ascherio A, Rimm EB, et al. A prospective cohort study of vasectomy and prostate cancer in US men. *JAMA.* 1993;269:873–877. doi:10.1001/jama.1993.03500070053028

16. D'Souza G, Kreimer AR, Viscidi R, et al. Case-control study of human papillomavirus and oropharyngeal cancer. *N Engl J Med.* 2007;356:1944–1956. doi:10.1056/NEJMoa065497

17. Singh H, Banipal R. Psychological distress in cancer patient during chemotherapy: a cross-sectional study. *J Clin Oncol.* 2016;34(26 Suppl):231. doi:10.1200/jco.2016.34.26_suppl.231

18. Rades D, Huttenlocher S, Dunst J, et al. Matched pair analysis comparing surgery followed by radiotherapy and radiotherapy alone for metastatic spinal cord compression. *J Clin Oncol.* 2010;28:3597–3604. doi:10.1200/JCO.2010.28.5635
19. Mok TS, Wu Y-L, Ahn M-J, et al. Osimertinib or platinum-pemetrexed in *EGFR* T790M–positive lung cancer. *N Eng J Med.* 2017;376:629–640. doi: 10.1056/NEJMoa1612674
20. Pignon J-P, le Maître A, Maillard E, Bourhis J. Meta-analysis of chemotherapy in head and neck cancer (MACH-NC): an update on 93 randomised trials and 17, 346 patients. *Radiother and Oncol.* 2009;92:4–14. doi:10.1016/j.radonc.2009.04.014

Section III Problem Set

CLINICAL TRIALS AND RETROSPECTIVE STUDIES

1. Design a case-control study to investigate whether alcohol intake of more than three drinks per week is associated with risk of breast cancer.

2. Design a prospective cohort study to investigate whether alcohol intake of more than three drinks per week is associated with risk of breast cancer.

3. Design a retrospective cohort study to investigate whether alcohol intake of more than three drinks per week is associated with risk of breast cancer.

4. A three-arm trial designed to compare the disease-free survival of patients who are randomly assigned to receive an investigational therapy (that has previously been tested in clinical trials), the standard of care, and the combination of the investigational therapy together with the standard of care is best categorized as which phase clinical trial?

5. A single-arm trial designed to evaluate the safety of an investigational therapy is best categorized as which phase clinical trial?

6. A new medical device to be used in breast cancer surgeries has been shown to be more effective than the previous standard of care. It is now cleared by the FDA and is considered the new standard of care. A large multi-institutional group is tracking outcomes and adverse events in patients who have received this device as standard of care. This trial is best categorized as which phase clinical trial?

7. Multiple randomized clinical trials have been carried out to compare the use of prophylactic cranial irradiation, following response to chemotherapy for patients with limited stage small-cell lung cancer. Many of the trials have conflicting results. What would be a method to pool the results of the previously conducted trials to determine the result of an analysis with all subjects from all of the previously conducted trials?

8. You are conducting a study to identify factors associated with the development of G3–5 toxicity in patients receiving chemotherapy for metastatic cancer. You have hypothesized that age, number of lines of previous treatment, nutritional status, and performance status are associated with risk of G3–5 toxicity. Based on previous clinical trials, you determine that the risk of G3–5 toxicity with chemotherapy is about 10% in your clinic population. A minimum of how many patients should be included in the analysis?

Section III Problem Set Solutions

CLINICAL TRIALS AND RETROSPECTIVE STUDIES

1. Take patients with breast cancer (cases) and compare them retrospectively to patients without breast cancer (controls), and see whether the groups differ in the percentage of patients who drink more than three alcoholic drinks per week.

2. Take a sample of patients who drink more than three alcoholic drinks per week and a sample of patients who do not drink alcohol or who drink three alcoholic drinks per week or less, and follow them prospectively to see whether risk of developing breast cancer differs between the two groups.

3. Take a sample of patients who drink more than three alcoholic drinks per week and compare their history to the history of patients who do not drink alcohol or who drink three alcoholic drinks per week or less retrospectively to see whether the groups differ in the incidence of lung cancer.

4. Phase III

5. Phase I

6. Phase IV

7. An individual patient data meta-analysis

8. The sample size should accommodate 10 G3–5 toxicity events per variable investigated in a regression analysis. You have set out to investigate four variables in this regression analysis. Thus, $10 \times 4 = 40$ G3–5 toxicities should be accommodated by the sample size. If you anticipate a rate of 10% G3–5 toxicity, you should plan to include at least 400 patients in the analysis.

   $n = 400$.

SELF-ASSESSMENT QUESTIONS AND ANSWERS

1. The percentage of patients with breast cancer who have a core needle biopsy and who have suspicious findings during screening or diagnostic mammogram (BIRADS 4–6) is described by:
   a. Sensitivity
   b. Specificity
   c. True positives
   d. Positive predictive value

2. Survival curves from a randomized clinical trial comparing immunotherapy to chemotherapy in metastatic non-small cell lung cancer (NSCLC) demonstrates a median survival with immunotherapy of 13 months. Median survival is defined as:
   a. The average survival time
   b. The time point at which 50% of the sample is alive on a conditional survival curve
   c. The median age of the surviving sample
   d. The median time to event in patients who experienced an event

3. In a sample from a normally distributed population, what is the probability of a value being within two standard deviations of the mean?
   a. 99%
   b. 95%
   c. 75%
   d. 68%

4. What is the 95% confidence interval for a mean Hgb of 10.5 with a standard deviation of 1.3 in a sample of 100 patients?
   a. 10.25–10.76
   b. 7.9–13.1
   c. 9.85–11.15
   d. 9.2–11.8

5. **Which method best describes a retrospective study designed to examine the association between vitamin D deficiency and the risk of developing breast cancer based on comparison of the health histories of patients with and without breast cancer?**

   a. Phase I clinical trial

   b. Longitudinal study

   c. Cohort study

   d. Case-control study

6. **Which statistical analysis should be used to compare overall survival between two groups while controlling for age, body mass index, and performance status?**

   a. Cox proportional hazards regression

   b. Linear regression

   c. Logistic regression

   d. Pearson correlation

7. **Which of the following effect size estimators involves survival models?**

   a. Relative risk

   b. Odds ratio

   c. Hazard ratio

   d. p-value

8. **A Pearson correlation analysis is used to calculate r^2. What is the meaning of r^2?**

   a. The degree to which one variable varies with the changes in the other variable

   b. The y intercept of the linear regression equation

   c. The strength of the linear relationship between two variables

   d. The correlation coefficient

9. **Which of the following tests is most appropriate to analyze the relationship between a nominal independent and nominal dependent variable?**

   a. t-test

   b. Linear regression

   c. Pearson correlation

   d. Chi-square

10. **Calculate the relative risk of metastatic breast cancer with positive axillary lymph node on physical exam in women with newly diagnosed breast cancer based on the data presented in the following 2 x 2 table:**

	Axillary Lymph Node Exam Negative	Axillary Lymph Node Exam Positive	Total
Metastatic breast cancer negative	240	100	340
Metastatic breast cancer positive	20	25	45
Total	260	125	385

Relative Risk =

a. 1.6

b. 2.6

c. .62

d. .385

11. **The null hypothesis that a hazard ratio = 1 should be tested by which of the following analysis:**
    a. Logistic regression
    b. Linear regression
    c. Cox proportional hazards regression
    d. Pearson correlation

12. **What is the power of a test?**
    a. The probability of accepting the null hypothesis when it is true
    b. The strength of the association between two variables
    c. The probability of rejecting the null hypothesis when it is not true
    d. The probability of rejecting the null hypothesis when it is true

13. **Which test is the most appropriate to compare overall survival between two groups in a randomized trial after adjusting for patient performance status and comorbid illness?**
    a. Cox proportional hazards regression
    b. *t*-test
    c. Log-rank test
    d. Chi-square test

14. **What is the range of values that includes 95% of the population given a mean of 1.5 and a standard deviation of .1?**

    a. 1.4–1.6

    b. 1.3–1.7

    c. 1.2–1.8

    d. 1.1–1.9

15. **Which of the following measures decreases as the sample size increases?**

    a. Variance

    b. Standard error of the mean

    c. Standard deviation

    d. Coefficient of determination

16. **What is the null hypothesis for a study designed to test whether high-dose radiation treatment for lung cancer is associated with an increased risk of pneumonitis?**

    a. There is a linear relationship between radiation dose and the risk of pneumonitis.

    b. Increased radiation dose is associated with increased risk of pneumonitis.

    c. Increased radiation dose is associated with decreased risk of pneumonitis.

    d. There is no association between radiation dose and risk of pneumonitis.

17. **Which method should be used to combine data from multiple selected studies to develop a conclusion that has a greater statistical power?**

    a. Repetitive analysis

    b. Correlation

    c. Meta-analysis

    d. Multiple linear regression

18. **What is the positive likelihood ratio of test with a sensitivity of 80% and specificity of 80%?**

    a. .25

    b. .50

    c. 1

    d. 4

19. Which of the following distributions give the probability of the occurrence of one of the two possible outcomes in a fixed number of trials?

   a. Normal

   b. Binomial

   c. Gaussian

   d. Poisson

20. Which of the following distributions give the probability of a specific number of occurrences of a rare event in an very large number of trials?

   a. Normal

   b. Binomial

   c. Gaussian

   d. Poisson

21. You are conducting a case-control study and have included a total of 150 patients with breast cancer and 300 patients without breast cancer. Of the 150 patients with breast cancer, 68 have used hormone replacement therapy in the past. Of the 300 patients without breast cancer, 90 have used hormone replacement therapy in the past. What is the appropriate effect size modifier and value for analysis of this data?

   a. OR = 1.93

   b. RR = 1.93

   c. OR = 1.53

   d. RR = 1.53

22. A new type of prostate imaging is being used to detect prostate cancer. The test is administered to 1,000 patients, 200 of whom you know to have the disease. The test was positive in 100 of the 200 patients with the disease and in 50 of the patient who do NOT have the disease. What is the specificity of this test?

   a. 50%

   b. 93.75%

   c. 88%

   d. 85%

23. **Which of the following is dependent upon the total number of positive test results in a sample?**

    a. Sensitivity

    b. Specificity

    c. Positive predictive value

    d. Negative predictive value

24. **Which is the most appropriate test to compare means of two non-normally distributed examples?**

    a. *t*-test

    b. Wilcoxon rank-sum test

    c. ANOVA

    d. Chi-square test

25. **Which phase of clinical trial is most appropriate to determine the best way to administer a new medication?**

    a. Phase I

    b. Phase II

    c. Phase III

    d. Phase IV

1. a) **Sensitivity**—The definition of sensitivity is the proportion of patients with a disease who test positive.

2. b) **The time point at which 50% of the sample is alive on a conditional survival curve**—The median survival must be calculated from a conditional survival curve (e.g., Kaplan–Meier curve) and represents the time point on that curve at which half of the patients are alive and have of the patients are dead.

3. b) **95%;** 68% of observations fall within on standard deviation of the mean, 95% of the observations fall within two standard deviations of the mean, and 99.7% of the observations fall within three standard deviations of the mean.

4. a) **10.25 to 10.76:**
   95% CI = mean +/− (1.96 × SEM)
   SEM = standard deviation/($\sqrt{100}$) = 1.3/10 = 0.13
   95% CI = 10.5 +/− (1.96 × 0.13) = 10.5 +/− 0.255 = 10.25–10.76

5. d) **Case-control study**—In a case-control study, the groups are defined on the basis of outcome (groups defined as patients with and without the outcome of breast cancer).

6. a) **Cox proportional hazards regression**—Cox proportional hazards regression analyzes time-to-event data and also accounts for the effect of covariates.

7. c) **Hazard ratio**—The ratio of the risk of the event over a certain period of time for different categories of covariates in a time-to-event analysis such as disease-free survival or overalls survival. Odds ratio and relative risk involve regression and chi-square analysis without a component of survival or time-to-event data. p-value is not an effect size estimate.

8. a) **The degree to which one variable varies with the changes in the other variable**—r^2, the coefficient of determination is the square of the correlation coefficient and explains how much one variable varies with changes in the other variable or the percent of variance explained by the model.

9. **d) Chi-square**—The chi-square test compares the relationship between two nominal variables.

10. **b) 2.6**—To start, rearrange the table with the test to label the rows and the result to label the columns, and with the positive result in the top row and left column and the negative result in the bottom row and the right column.

	Metastatic Breast Cancer Positive	Metastatic Breast Cancer Negative	Total
Axillary lymph node positive	25	100	125
Axillary lymph node negative	20	240	260
Total	340	45	385

Relative risk = $((a/(a + b)/c/(c + d)) = (25/125)/(20/260) = .2/.077 = 2.6$

11. **c) Cox proportional hazards regression**—The cox proportional hazards model produces hazard ratios.

12. **c) The probability of rejecting the null hypothesis when it is not true**—The power of a test is the probability of detecting a difference that exists. It can be stated as the probability of rejecting the null hypothesis when it is not true.

13. **a) Cox proportional hazards regression**—Cox regression analysis can be used to compare survival curves after adjusting for covariates.

14. **b) 1.3 to 1.7**—68% of the observations fall within on standard deviation of the mean, 95% of the observations fall within two standard deviations of the mean, and 99.7% of the observations fall within three standard deviations of the mean.

15. **b) Standard error of the mean**—SEM = standard deviation/$\sqrt{n}$. Thus, mathematically, as n increases, SEM decreases.

16. **d) Radiation dose is not associated with risk of pneumonitis**—The null hypothesis $H_0: d = 0$.

17. **c) Meta-analysis**—A meta-analysis is a statistical analysis that combines the data of multiple scientific studies or clinical trials. Aggregation of information from multiple smaller studies into one large meta-analysis

allows for increased statistical power to detect the effect being examined. A meta-analysis also includes a sample with overall greater diversity among subjects.

18. d) 4—Positive likelihood ratio = Sensitivity/(1 – Specificity) = 80%/20% = .80/.20 = 4.

19. b) **Binomial**—In a binomial distribution, each event has two possible outcomes with a fixed number of n trials. One of the possible outcomes is considered a success, and one of the possible outcomes is considered a failure.

20. d) **Poisson**—The Poisson distribution addresses the probability of a rare outcome within an interval of time, space, distance, area, and/or volume in a very large or infinite number of trials.

21. a) **OR = 1.93**

The 2 × 2 table is constructed as follows:

	Positive Breast Cancer	No Breast Cancer
Use of HRT	68	90
No use of HRT	82	210

As this is a case-control study, the odds ratio is the most appropriate effect size modifier.

$OR = (a/c)/(b/d) = ad/bc = (68 \times 210)/(90 \times 82) = 14280/7380 = 1.93$

22. b) **93.75%**

	Presence of Disease		
	Positive	Negative	Total
Test result			
Positive	100	50	150
Negative	100	750	850
Total	200	800	1000

Specificity = $d/(d + b)$ = 750/800 = 93.75%

23. c) **Positive predictive value**—For a given test administered to a population with the following results:

	Presence of Disease		
	Positive	**Negative**	**Total**
Test result			
Positive	*a*	*b*	*a + b*
Negative	*b*	*d*	*c + d*
Total	*a + c*	*b + d*	*a + b + c + d*

Positive predictive value (PPV) = $a/(a + b)$. $(a + b)$ is the total number of positive tests.

24. **b) Wilcoxon rank-sum test**—The Wilcoxon rank-sum test is a nonparametric test similar to the independent t-test used to compare the means of two independent samples that may not be normally distributed.

25. **a) Phase I**—A Phase I trial often addresses the best way to administer a new medication (e.g., determining the maximum-tolerated dose (MTD) for the new medication).

Index

Printed in the United States
By Bookmasters